Exploring Rural Medicine

EXPLORING RURAL MEDICINE

CURRENT ISSUES AND CONCEPTS

BARBARA P. YAWN
ANGELINE BUSHY
ROY A. YAWN
EDITORS

SAGE Publications
International Educational and Professional Publisher
Thousand Oaks   London   New Delhi

For information address:

SAGE Publications, Inc.
2455 Teller Road
Thousand Oaks, California 91320

SAGE Publications Ltd.
6 Bonhill Street
London EC2A 4PU
United Kingdom

SAGE Publications India Pvt. Ltd.
M-32 Market
Greater Kailash I
New Delhi 110 048 India

Printed in the United States of America

Library of Congress Cataloging-in-Publication Data

Main entry under title:

Exploring rural medicine: current issues and concepts / edited by
    Barbara P. Yawn, Angeline Bushy, Roy A. Yawn.
        p. cm.
    Includes bibliographical references and index.
    ISBN 0-8039-4851-4 (cl). — ISBN 0-8039-4852-2 (pb)
    1. Medicine, Rural—United States. I. Yawn, Barbara. II. Bushy,
Angeline. III. Yawn, Roy A.
RA771.5.E95 1994
362.1'0425—dc20   93-27090

94 95 96 97 10 9 8 7 6 5 4 3 2 1

Sage Production Editor: Diane S. Foster

Contents

8. Common Mental Health Problems

LAWRENCE P. PETERSON

19. Making Your Practice Palatable for Your Patients: Cultural Competency

BARBARA P. YAWN and ANGELINE BUSHY,
with KATHY DUBBELS, PELAGE "MIKE" SNESRUD,
and CAROLE E. HILL

20. Ethics Dilemmas in Rural Practice

ANGELINE BUSHY and J. RANDALL RAUH

For our fathers
Louis O. Padgett, 1922–1965
Levie "Pete" Yawn, 1927–1992

And our sons
Nathan Yawn
Peter Yawn

Barbara Yawn
Roy Yawn

To my husband Jack
and
my daughter Andrea Dacyl

Angeline Bushy

Notice

The editors, authors, and publisher of this book have made every effort to assure that the drug indications and dose schedules cited are accurate and consistent with currently accepted standards at the time of publication. Because of the rapidly changing nature of medical practice, readers are advised to refer to the product information sheet and other current sources for each drug they use to assure that changes have not been made in the indications for use, contraindications, or recommended doses.

Preface

The practice of medicine in rural America is different from medical practice in urban or suburban America. Rural physicians are called upon to care for a broad range of problems with a limited number of available technological, nursing, and consultant resources. Because of the lack of resources, physicians need to have knowledge about some unique topics not generally covered in textbooks of medicine or family practice. Seldom do physicians have access to practical details about medical management for rural problems such as stabilization of farm accident victims, preservation of a severed limb for transport, therapeutic approaches to socially isolated rural women, resources for the rural chemically dependent, or techniques to develop alternative practice styles compatible with specific rural needs. This book is designed to cover some of the topics needed by rural practitioners and not usually found in any textbook. Although it will be impossible to cover every topic potentially useful to the rural physician, this book presents information in a variety of practice areas as well as information important to the survival of a rural physician in the rapidly changing regulatory environment.

We believe this text will be a unique reference for the care of individuals with specific rural problems, for prevention techniques tailored to promote health in rural communities, and for information to support a successful rural practice. Each chapter is written by practitioners with vast experience with rural patients. Some have practiced in rural areas; other serve as consultants to large numbers of rural practitioners and their patients. All the authors have a respect for and appreciation of the extra burden carried by those who choose a rural practice, and they understand the need for all health care disciplines to work together..

BARBARA P. YAWN, MD, MS
ANGELINE BUSHY, PhD, RN
ROY A. YAWN, MD
—EDITORS

1
■ ■ ■

Rural Medical Practice:
Present and Future

BARBARA P. YAWN

Introduction

Until recently, rural medical practice was ignored by most medical educators, health policy planners, physicians in training, and the media. A few policy groups like the Robert Wood Johnson Foundation and some medical schools including those in the states of Washington and North Carolina recognized the importance of a unique style of training for rural physicians. But most rural physicians currently practicing grew up in rural areas and simply returned to communities similar to those of their youth. Severe shortages of obstetrical and primary care providers in the deep South have forced some states to examine rural medical issues but few have found solutions. Health care reform, primarily cost containment efforts, has renewed the focus on rural medical practice. It has become obvious that the disparities in economic resources and numbers and types of health care providers, and the higher risk rural population are not amenable to transplanted urban solutions. This chapter outlines some of the economic, demographic, and health characteristics that make rural populations and their health care needs different from those of the urban areas. Recommendations for the prioritization of required services based on the population density is presented. Finally, an overview of the current proposals for reform of the health care delivery system are presented with a short discussion of their potential impact on rural medical practice.

Characteristics of Rural Areas

Rural can mean many different things. Often the definitions of rurality are similar to those for art or beauty or pornography—I cannot define it but I will know it when I see it. However, the government has chosen to define *rural* by making it synonymous with nonmetropolitan:

> Rural areas are all parts of the country located outside of a metropolitan statistical area (MSA). An MSA is any area containing a city with a population of at least 50,000 or an urban area with a population of at least 50,000 or a total metropolitan population of at least 100,000. MSAs are defined as entire counties. An MSA includes the county containing the main city and other counties having strong economic and social ties to the central county. (American Hospital Association [AHA], 1992)

This definition is very misleading for large counties with a single large population center. Recently the concept of "frontier area" has been added to identify those areas with extremely sparsely populated areas, defined as less than six residents per square mile (Elison, 1986).

"Rural" may be better defined by the economics, social structure, and demographics of an area than by its population density or proximity to an urban center. Overall, rural residents tend to be more conservative, more self-directed, less well educated, older, poorer, more likely to be self-employed or unemployed, and more likely to have acute and chronic illnesses. Rural areas are more likely to be economically dependent on a single industry—farming, mining, forestry, or a manufacturing plant. All rural-based industries have shown slow growth or even losses over the past decade. Most rural areas of the country lost population between the 1980 and 1990 census (AHA, 1992).

"Rural" can also be defined by health care needs and resources. Rural residents are more likely to be uninsured or underinsured, and part of an intact family with a single wage earner and therefore less likely to be eligible for Medicaid. In the past, rural medical providers have received lower reimbursements for Medicare and Medicaid and often for private insurance coverage. On most measures of health, rural residents fall behind urban people: more days with restricted activity, more injuries, more acute illnesses, and more chronic conditions (Office of Technology Assessment, 1990). Part of the difference is accounted for by the high concentration of elderly residents in rural areas, and the greater proportion of rural people employed in hazardous occupations such as farming or mining. But overall, rural residents have lower mortality rates.

Rural areas have fewer physicians, nurses, and allied health professionals. However, the overall averages obscure differences between rural sections of the country with severe shortages and others with sufficient providers of one type or another. For example, the rural northeastern part of the United States has 303 physicians per 100,000 residents, the rural west 235 per 100,000, and the rural south only 184 per 100,000. These numbers reflect the gains in numbers of providers over the past 5 years in most rural areas, with the exceptions of losses in rural Florida (3.8 physicians per 100,000 residents) and frontier Wyoming (17.6 per 100,000) (Office of Technology Assessment, 1990). Future projections for availability of providers must consider that 13% of practicing rural physicians are over the age of 65 compared to only 9% of practicing urban physicians who are over 65. In the 1980s the supply of rural nurses increased, perhaps due to the large number of women over 35 to 40 who returned to nursing during the farming crisis. Numbers of midlevel practitioners have not increased significantly (AHA, 1992).

Most rural areas have decreased access to advanced medical technology. However, the use of mobile technology has left few areas without any access to obstetrical ultrasound, computerized tomographic scans, and even magnetic resonance imaging and angiography (Christianson & Moscovice, 1993). Rural hospitals generally have more expenses than revenues and many have closed. Others have become acute care facilities with expanded outpatient services. The ratio of hospital beds to population is equal in urban and rural areas. However, the rural population tends to have more admissions and shorter hospital stays (Office of Technology Assessment, 1990). This may be due to admissions that are required to complete testing and stabilization of patients who cannot travel back and forth to the hospital or physicians' offices easily.

With the deluge of medical reporting in magazines, newspapers, and television programs, the rural population has increased its medical expectations and its outshopping behavior. It is not unusual for rural residents, particularly the more affluent, to bypass local medical facilities and providers to seek essentially identical services in large urban centers. The use of visiting specialists has helped to reverse this trend in communities where the specialists come to communities at the request of local providers (AHA, 1992).

Considering all the seemingly negative factors, how close are we coming to providing the necessary medical care for rural residents? The answer is not a simple one. As anyone who has traveled around the United States knows, rural areas are extremely diverse. Can some general needs of the frontier areas of Wyoming and the more densely populated but rural areas of New England be combined and prioritized into categories or levels of care?

Have Rural Medical Needs Been Defined?

It is unreasonable to assume that rural health care will ever look exactly like urban health care. Indeed it may not be appropriate merely to impose urban needs for providers on the rural areas. Two studies have helped to identify necessary services for rural areas. Both are useful when examining the services that currently exist and those that may be important to institute. The Washington Rural Health Care Commission defined bands or levels of service necessary for the rural areas (see Table 1.1). The first band contains services most critical to people's survival or most often utilized (emergency and primary care services). The second band is basic diagnostic support services; the third band is an essential core of basic acute care and home health services. The fourth band is for community-based care of chronic conditions and the fifth band defines services that help residents in larger populated rural areas stay within the community for care (Washington Rural Health Care Commission, 1989).

Utah has defined tiers of services specifically for frontier areas. The types of services recommended are based on the population of the area (Figure 1.1) (Elison, 1986).

The table and figure are a useful way to assess the needs of your community or the adequacy of resources of a county you are considering as your new home and practice site. In addition to an assessment of the community's needs, it is helpful take a personal assessment and to evaluate your ability to deal with the aspects of practice style that are different in a rural community compared to urban practices.

text continued on p. 7

Table 1.1 Basic Health Services for Rural Areas

Band 1: Prevent death, disability, serious illness
    24-hour emergency medical services (first responder/EMT)
        stabilization
        communications
        air-to-ground ambulance transport
    essential public health services
        environmental services, protection and monitoring
        personal health services and monitoring
    primary care
        routine health maintenance
        prevention
        care for acute conditions
        prenatal care
    mental health services
        crisis intervention

Band 2: Necessary support services for Band 1
    diagnostic services
        simple X rays, fluoroscopy, ultrasound
        laboratory for blood chemistries, hematology, urines, and bacteriology

Band 3: Short-term inpatient and home health services
    home health services
        visiting nurse
        medical services
        durable equipment
    selected acute short-term hospital services
        common conditions—pneumonia, gastroenteritis, accidents
        childbirth, uncomplicated

Band 4: Community-based care for chronic conditions
    mental health services
        evaluation
        consultation
        therapy including counseling
    long-term care services
        community-based home care services
        supervised living, respite care, and day care
        skilled and intermediate nursing homes
    substance abuse and chemical dependency services
        counseling and intervention
        treatment referral

Band 5: Other services
    dental care
    vision and hearing care
    hospice care

SOURCE: Washington Rural Health Care Commission (1986).

Population/ Service Area	Emergency Medical Services	Primary Care	Specialty Care	Hospitalization
Fewer than 500 persons	First responder EMT	Intermittent MLP or MD by appointment; Satellite/part-time clinic EMT supervision via telecommunication and written protocol	Referral	Referral
500-900 persons	EMT First responder network in outlying areas	Full-time MLP or part-time MD Arrangement for emergency coverage and EMT supervision	Referral or periodic arrangement in the community	Referral
900-1,500 persons	EMT First responder network	Full-time MD or MLP, or combination full- and part-time group practice Emergency coverage and EMT supervision	Referral or periodic arrangement in the community	Referral and in-firmary model
1,500-4,000+ persons	EMT First responder network	Small group practice: combination MD and/or MLP; medical specialists (MD/ MLP; IM, PED or OB, CNM as determined by community need Emergency coverage and EMT supervision	On-site full-time regularly scheduled clinic within primary care practice Referral	Small community hospital or in-firmary Referral

Figure 1.1. Recommended Health Services by Size of Community

SOURCE: Elison (1986).
NOTE: CNM = certified nurse midwife; EMT = emergency medical technician; IM = internist; MD = medical doctor; MLP = midlevel practitioner; OB = obstetrician; PED = pediatrician.

How Is Rural Practice Different?

Rural practice is different from urban practice and different from the practices most of us learned while in residency training. Family practice residencies are often urban hospital-based programs using specialists as preceptors. The patients we see during our training are from the tip of the disease iceberg. They come from the 1 to 9 per 1,000 people who not only become ill each month but who are hospitalized or seen by a consultant (Figure 1.2). In rural practice you will see the 250 per 1,000 who visit physicians each month; and you are likely to be aware of many of the 500 more who are ill or injured but who do not seek medical care directly. The needs of those you do see are often very different from those patients your training taught you to treat. Most family practice residents can manage a cardiac arrest but have trouble with an ingrown toenail or simple back strain. Much of the daily treatment of primary care problems is learned on the job from colleagues and our patients.

In rural practice consultants are usually in distant sites requiring telephone consultation. Like the preferences most of us developed for certain preceptors, teachers, and consultants during our training, most rural physicians will develop a network of consultants who know and respect the skills of the rural physician and the health care community and hospital. Until those networks are developed it can be very frustrating to work within the framework of limited equipment and testing capabilities. Mobile technology services can be invaluable as can the services of a visiting pathologist or radiologist.

Most rural physicians will have admitting privileges in at least one rural hospital. The demands for physician time to serve on hospital committees and provide administrative support to the community health boards can be very intense. With a limited hospital staff, developing multiple competencies in the staff and finding alternatives to physician membership on all committees is necessary. If you have several visiting specialists with only courtesy privileges it may be possible to have some hospital meetings on days when they are present to allow them to attend as medical staff representatives.

Unlike some of our urban colleagues, rural physicians continue to be held in high esteem. Perhaps it is the fact that our rural patients recognize the hours we work, or that they become person-

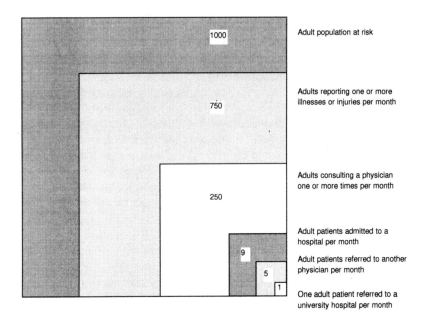

Figure 1.2. Monthly Prevalence Estimate of Illness in the Community
SOURCE: "Ecology of Medical Care," by K. L. White, T. F. Williams, & B. G. Greenberg, 1961, *New Engl J Med, 265*, 885-892.

ally acquainted with our families, or merely have greater need for each of us individually. Rural physicians enjoy great respect and prestige in their communities. Although the opportunities for professional growth may seem limited, most rural physicians have unlimited opportunities to develop special areas of expertise and interest. Whether it is cardiology, emergency medicine, patient education, child abuse prevention, or preventive medicine, it is unlikely that any other provider will be there to prevent your choice of special interest practices or the development of expertise in that field.

Unlike many of our urban colleagues, few rural primary care physicians can limit their practices to only one or a few areas that we find most rewarding or feel most competent to handle. Rural practice requires broad-based knowledge and skills. It is not unusual to go from a minor trauma case in the emergency department to the delivery room to the family of an elderly dying patient. You are likely to be the local nursing home director, the school health physician, and the resource for patient education. It is impossible to be expert in each of these fields. Rural physicians must learn to deal with levels of uncertainty that might prompt their urban colleagues to obtain a formal or informal consultation. The use of such consultations is often infeasible and is probably excessive. Learning to live with the risk of being wrong 1 or 2 times in every 10,000 tension headaches is not an unreasonable risk considering the risks our patients take in driving on the highway to get to our offices.

During training or in urban practices, physicians are often sheltered from alternative care providers. Rural people who define *health* as the ability to work are willing to use any services they believe will help them return to their usual activities. Almost one third of the nation's population makes at least one visit each year to a health care professional other than a physician or dentist (Thorp, 1992). In rural areas this fraction jumps to 40%. More than 5% visit chiropractors, about 14% visit nurses, 12% visit optometrists, 2% see podiatrists, and 6% consult others such as lay counselors, ministers, and faith or herbal healers. The rural resident does not always share the physician's world view that 20th-century technology-based medicine is the exclusive, comprehensive health care modality. Many of the alternative practitioners and their training and expertise may be unfamiliar to the physician. It is important to find out who else provides care in your community, what services they offer, and what their history is in the community. Contradicting the advice of the local chiropractor who has lived and worked in the community during the short tenure of the past nine local physicians is unwise and often counterproductive. Patience, individual patient education, and proof of your community concern and abilities will make new ideas more palatable and more likely to be considered.

No discussion of the differences in rural practice is complete without at least a mention of the community itself. Unlike our urban colleagues, we live, work, eat, and play in the same schools, churches, parks, and neighborhoods as do our patients. Often our children and spouses compete for the same jobs or academic and athletic recognition as those of our patients and their children. Not every physician is able to accept the same people as patients and close friends. The aspirations your neighbors have for their children may be very different from the aspirations you have for your children, making even discussion of children difficult.

Physicians who have never lived in a small rural community may find the available sources of recreation and relaxation very different from those they enjoyed as children and students. Although a metropolitan area with other resources may be only a few hours away, the time constraints of practice may make travel difficult. New physicians may delay social activities until they are more comfortable in their new practices. The delay is understandable but if it is too long you may not truly integrate into your new neighborhood and community.

Rural practice has been evolving and changing since World War II, when physicians found they suddenly had the tools and resources to cure as well as to diagnose many diseases. Technology, mass media, and better training of all physicians have improved medical care in urban and rural America. But many people talk about the need for cataclysmic change in health care delivery systems. Rural medicine will not be left unchanged. But special attention must be paid to the potential impact of proposed changes on rural health care. They are unlikely to be the same or even similar to the impact on urban health care.

What Is the Future of Rural Medicine?

Health care reform will affect the practice of medicine in all parts of the United States, but the rural areas may have unique issues that deserve special solutions. In order to understand what some of those unique issues may be it is important to understand the general concepts of health care reform that are being proposed.

To the new student of reform the current proposals sound like "word salad." Understanding these proposals requires you to understand the terms. We can then put the terms or concepts together to analyze the potential impact on rural practice.

Health Care Reform Terminology

Managed care implies that the overall care a patient receives is limited by someone other than the patient. The "management" may be from a third-party payor who requires prior authorization, determines which services will be reimbursed under the insurance plan, or which physician or consultant is an acceptable part of the patient's care options. This is not necessarily synonymous with **coordinated care**, which provides services to oversee and coordinate the total health care needs of a person, usually with chronic conditions.

Integrated service networks are often modeled on the health maintenance organization (HMO) concept. This may be a group of providers who are independent practitioners working together or a group of providers who are employees of a network much like HMOs such as Group Health or Kaiser Permanente. The network contracts with purchasers to provide services, usually for a capitation fee. The providers in the group may be salaried or paid on a fee-for-service basis. Several large urban-based integrated service networks exist. These networks are usually for profit, limit the enrollees to those with low health care needs, and serve high density population areas.

Guaranteed access includes several concepts. Most often it refers to financial access. Each person is to have some type of financial plan (usually insurance coverage) that pays for medical care. Exactly what care is covered and what personal responsibility in the form of copayments and deductibles is incorporated vary greatly, and may not even be discussed. Some plans require ethnic or cultural access, requiring interpreters to be available at all times. Geographic access is seldom addressed or specifically defined.

Managed competition is the reform concept du jour. First proposed by the Jackson Hole Group of self-designated policy and reform experts, it has been used, abused, and reinterpreted by almost every reform effort in the past 2 years. In its original form, managed competition called for large integrated service networks to be developed to provide care for 350,000 to 500,000 people. They would compete for service contracts that require certain basic benefits to be covered. The competition is to be based on price and quality of services. The quality is to be determined on the basis of "outcome" studies of varying services and patient satisfaction. The Jackson Hole Group has said that they do not believe that managed competition will be feasible in rural areas. This has led to a new term, "managed collaboration."

Managed collaboration is specifically designed for rural areas. This allows rural integrated service networks to develop with the collaboration of rural providers. Because the population numbers are inadequate to support competing networks, the providers are required to collaborate to lower costs. The same type of quality data would be required from the collaborating networks as from the competing networks.

Outcome studies have become an important research tool. These studies look at the outcomes of various treatment strategies for a particular problem or diagnosis, such as benign prostatic hypertrophy (BPH). The studies compare the outcomes (rates of urinary incontinence, impotence, and postoperative hemorrhage) of various treatments for BPH (surgery, medication, or observation). Few outcomes are easily measured using currently available data such as insurance claim forms.

Global budgets would place a limit on health care expenditures. In some cases the limits are set for all health care expenditures including out-of-pocket expenses like aspirin and elective cosmetic surgery; but other proposed global budgets include only those services for which coverage would be required by insurance programs. Most global budgets allow for some increase in health care expenditures over the next 5 years.

Practice parameters are guidelines that would tell a physician what type of testing and treatment is appropriate or required for a particular complaint or diagnosis. Many practice parameters have been developed by specialty societies and consensus groups. Few are based on sound research or medical data and even fewer have been tested. The parameters are intended to decrease regional variation in care and to lower costs.

Expanded rights to practice are considered to be necessary to assure that rural areas will have some practitioners. Usually the reform plans discuss allowing nurse practitioners and physicians' assistants to practice medicine without direct supervision. Other changes would allow optometrists and other types of practitioners to have expanded privileges to prescribe drugs and to treat certain conditions.

Education of rural providers is recognized as an area that is ripe for change. Several of the reform programs call for expansion of loan repayment programs for rural providers. New education programs will allow or require part of the physician's training experience to occur in rural practice sites.

Health insurance purchasing cooperatives (HIPCs) are large collections of people or employers who band together to buy insurance at lower costs. They may be run by governments or private groups.

Data systems are believed to be available that will yield comprehensive information about services provided, the cost of those services, who paid for the services, and the outcomes of the services. These data systems will provide the basis for a region-wide computerized system.

What Would the
New System Look Like?

A mandated set of benefits will probably be defined at the federal level to be provided by the integrated service networks and all other providers. All individuals and employers will share the cost of health insurance through new taxes, with subsidies for the poor. Coverage will be purchased through health insurance purchasing cooperatives. The HIPCs will contract with integrated service networks or other groups of providers. The networks or groups of providers are paid by risk adjusted capitation, although individual providers within the plans could be paid using a variety of different methods. The HIPC pays an amount equal to the cost of the lowest benefit plan; consumers may choose to pay extra for a higher cost plan with more benefits. States will supervise the HIPCs to allow some flexibility for the development of innovative regional plans. Global budgets allowing total health care expenses to increase at or slightly above the rate of inflation will be set by the federal government. If the state or regional programs do not control costs, the federal government can set or freeze fees (price controls). Medicaid is eliminated and rolled into the HIPCs, but the elderly would continue to receive coverage under Medicare for at least the first few years (Christianson & Moscovice, 1993).

The system requires a large new bureaucracy to manage all the elements. States must develop mechanisms to facilitate and oversee the functioning of the HIPCs, assure that data on quality of care and outcomes is gathered and distributed, and that costs are contained. The federal government will have to do the same things at the federal level, comparing not just HIPCs and integrated service networks but also the data on costs and outcomes from the individual states. Federal expenditures will have to be monitored to assure that all states are staying within the budget. If a state is unable to serve its bureaucratic function, the federal government will have to assume that task as well. Although national concerns are important, it is likely that rural providers will have more local concerns.

Practice Organization Concerns

At this time there are many more questions than answers about the effects of health care reform on rural medical practice. Rural physicians should be cognizant of the relevant questions and concerns, so that they can be effective advocates for the provision of excellent medical care. Rural physicians should be able to converse knowledgeably about health care reform with patients, colleagues, influential community members and officials, and legislators.

If managed competition does not work in rural areas, how will managed collaboration work? Will rural providers be able to form the necessary networks? Currently several barriers exist to the formation of such networks by rural providers: antitrust laws, lack of financial capital and expertise to develop the administrative services required, and often a lack of desire to participate in and recognition of the value of such networks. Because many of the networks appear to be similar to HMOs or other large insurance programs, will the urban-based plans organize rural networks before the rural providers have a chance to do so?

Who will be included in the rural networks and what services will be required in the basic or minimal benefit packages? Currently 40% of rural residents use alternative care providers at least once per year. Will the programs be required to incorporate these other providers? What do we include in the data set for quality measures of herbal healers, for instance?

What will happen to people and providers in areas where no networks are formed or where local providers refuse to join networks? If two or three networks come into an area, will a provider need to join all of them? How will this affect the administrative burden of the local provider?

Could networks be developed that improve the practice conditions for rural providers? Could urban groups provide coverage for rural physicians, allowing them more time off and local continuing medical education? Would rural hospitals and physicians join together to develop a single health care service, avoiding duplication of laboratory and radiology facilities? Can more urban-based specialty services be brought to the rural areas, stemming the flow of rural residents to larger urban facilities?

Can practice parameters and guidelines be modified to account for the primary care patients seen in rural areas? Primary care patients typically are seen early in the disease process rather than later in the process, which is the perspective of the subspecialists who write the parameters.

Would the parameters allow patients to make choices and assume risks as they often choose to do in rural and remote areas?

Reimbursement Concerns

If networks are paid on a capitation basis, will rural providers be required to share in the risk that the medical care provided will cost more than the available resources? Can sufficiently large networks be established in rural and frontier areas to allow capitation to cover all the financial risks of providing care to those groups? With smaller groups of older people with more chronic illnesses and younger people in more hazardous jobs, the risk of needing health care is higher but the ability to spread the risk smaller.

What will be the incentives for rural physicians, especially primary care providers, to become effective "gatekeepers" by limiting referrals to more expensive specialists? Will fee schedules be similar to those currently in existence, with higher fees paid to subspecialists and east and west coast urban physicians?

Recruitment and Retention Concerns

How will rural physicians react to the increased oversight and intrusion into their practices that will inevitably occur under any of the currently proposed reform packages? Can rural physicians respond to the increased requests for data about their practices and their patients?

Can the physicians who currently choose to practice in rural areas be retained under the new systems? Can the system be modified to assure that those providers are retained? Will a new generation of rural providers be recruited? Perhaps the changes will allow a different type of person to become a rural physician—one who is less independent, one who appreciates the direct support of urban groups that provide regular locum tenens service. It would be unfortunate if the reform programs choose to remake rural practice to fit the public health service model of short-term providers or to fit the triage model of limited service (or limited education) providers who dispense only minor care or stabilization services.

Summary

Rural medicine and rural physicians are different from their urban counterparts. For energetic, creative physicians great opportunities exist in rural areas: opportunities to continue to provide excellent rural health care and to mold health care reform to fit the needs and desires of people in rural America.

References

American Hospital Association (AHA). (1992). *Environmental assessment for rural hospitals, 1992.* Chicago: Author.

Christianson, J., & Moscovice, I. (1993). *Health care reform for rural areas.* Minneapolis: University of Minnesota, Rural Health Research Center.

Elison, G. (1986). Frontier areas: Problems for delivery of health care services. *Rural Health Care, 8*(5), 1-3.

Office of Technology Assessment. (1990). *Health care in rural America.* Washington, DC: Government Printing Office.

Thorp, J. P. (1992). Alternative practitioners and rural health care. In A. Bushy (Ed.), *Rural nursing* (pp. 79-92). Newbury Park, CA: Sage.

Washington Rural Health Care Commission. (1989). *A report to the legislature on rural health care in the state of Washington.* Olympia, WA: Author.

White, K. L., Williams, T. F., & Greenberg, B. G. (1961). Ecology of medical care. *New England Journal of Medicine, 265,* 888-892.

Recommended Reading

Yawn, B. P., & Yawn, R. A. (1992). Health care reform in Minnesota: Implications for the rural physician. *Minnesota Medicine, 75,* 32-36.

Yawn, B. P., Jacott, W. P., & Yawn, R. A. (1993). MinnesotaCare (HealthRight): Myths and miracles. *Journal of the American Medical Association, 269,* 511-515.

2

■ ■ ■

Labor and Delivery Crises:

Rural Solutions

CHARLES S. FIELD

BARBARA P. YAWN

Introduction

Delivering babies is one of the most stimulating, satisfying, and anxiety provoking events in the practice of rural medicine. Through years of careful observation and study we have learned the warning signs and symptoms associated with many obstetrical catastrophes. We have standardized risk assessment systems and tests to warn us of potential preeclampsia, gestational diabetes, preterm labor, and intrauterine growth retardation. With the help of obstetrical, perinatal, and neonatal colleagues in tertiary care centers we can evaluate, treat, and manage most of the obstetrical problems in our own hospitals and offices. When necessary we can refer in a timely nonemergent or controlled emergent manner.

But some obstetrical problems happen with less warning and at a time that leaves the rural practitioner with few options for transfer. Most of these occur at the time of labor and delivery. Some require immediate action, leaving little time for consultation. It is these urgent or emergent situations occurring at or near delivery that we will discuss in this chapter.

Each situation will begin with a short presentation of a case that is the synopsis of several cases that most rural family physicians, nurse midwives, and obstetricians have faced. This chapter will discuss the birthing process; the next chapter discusses the care of the infant immediately after birth.

Dysfunctional Labor

Case Report

Mrs. Jones, a 25-year-old married school teacher who is gravida 2, para 0, aborta 1 (a spontaneous unexplained abortion about 18 months ago), entered the hospital 6 hours ago. History shows a normal prenatal course, a negative hepatitis B surface antigen, and negative Rh factor. She received Rhogam at 28 weeks gestation.

On admission, the blood pressure is 113/68, fetal heart rate is 136, and the fetal head is in the right lower quadrant. The infant is active by palpation, with a vertex presentation and a fundal height of 37 centimeters. The cervix is 4 to 5 centimeters dilated, 1 centimeter thick, and soft. The head is at station 0 to -1. Contractions are occurring every 4 to 5 minutes, and are judged to be of good quality.

One hour ago the nurse heard two episodes of decelerations while monitoring the fetal heartbeat during and after contractions. Electronic fetal monitoring is begun and reveals no further decelerations with good beat to beat variability and return to the baseline. The night nurse coming on the next shift is new and was hired for her intensive care unit experience. You decide to come to stay in the hospital.

The night nurse reports that Mrs. Jones is 6 centimeters dilated, and the rest of exam is unchanged since admission. Contractions continue to occur every 3 to 4 minutes, duration 60 seconds, and are painful for the patient. The fetal monitoring strip reveals no abnormalities.

Diagnosis and Treatment

Is this a dysfunctional labor? You confirm that Mrs. Jones's cervical dilation is 6 cm, a progression of only 2 cm in the 6 hours since admission. However, your examination also shows that the cervix is thin and the baby's head is at station +1. With reassurance and ambulation, the patient becomes more comfortable and in 1 hour cervical dilation reaches 8 cm. She delivers a healthy infant 4 hours

Table 2.1 Definition of Dysfunctional Labor

	Nulliparous	*Multiparous*
Latent phase	> 21 hours	> 14 hours
Active phase		
dilation	< 1.2 cm/hr	< 1.5 cm/hr
no change for	> 2 hr	> 2 hr
Deceleration phase	> 3 hr	> 1 hr
Descent	< 1 cm/hr	< 2 cm/hr
	OR	OR
	no descent > 1 hr	no descent > ½ hr

later after pushing for 45 minutes. The placenta is delivered intact and the midline episiotomy is repaired without difficulty.

Although cervical dilation seemed to progress slowly, cervical effacement and descent of the presenting part continued during the first 6 hours after admission. This was not a dysfunctional labor but might have been treated as such if only the single variable of cervical dilation was considered. Recording the information on a labor curve prevented the use of oxytocin or an unnecessary cesarean section.

Discussion

The diagnosis of dysfunctional labor patterns (DLP) accounts for 45% to 60% of all cesarean sections. The evaluation of a labor pattern is most easily done by graphic representation of the progress of labor. Standardized preprinted Friedman labor curves are available for routine use. In many rural hospitals, there are no full-time labor and delivery staff nurses. Because rotating nurses may have less obstetrical experience it is necessary to have specific protocols for evaluation and treatment of DLP. Even in busy labor and delivery suites, written protocols facilitate prompt, thorough, and appropriate responses to any labor pattern. Protocols should include the definition of DLP (Table 2.1), the completion of a labor curve (Figure 2.1) on all women who deliver in more than 1 hour, and guidelines for contacting the attending physicians. Without this graphic reminder it may be difficult for nurses and physicians to be appropriately patient or active in the management of "slow" labors.

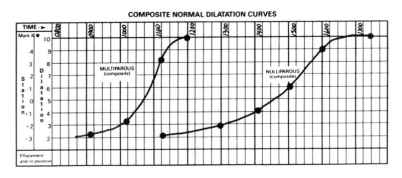

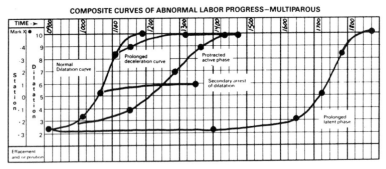

Figure 2.1. Labor Curve

SOURCE: Copyright 1975, 1979, 1986 by Hollister, Inc. Permission to reproduce this copyrighted material has been granted by the owner, Hollister Incorporated.

The three primary causes of DLP are abnormalities of the fetus, abnormalities of the birth canal, and insufficient or abnormal uterine contractions. Each potential cause must be assessed before appropriate therapy can be undertaken.

Abnormalities of the fetus are most likely to result in failure of the presenting part to descend; a large or structurally abnormal head, unflexed head and neck, and unrecognized twins are considerations. Most of these possibilities can be assessed with an ultrasound examination (if available on site) or with a single feto-gram (X ray).

Abnormalities of the birth canal may include abnormalities of the rigid or semirigid structures of the pelvis. The most severe of these may be noted during clinical pelvimetry. The use of X-ray pelvimetry has become unpopular but is occasionally useful. Inadequate size of the maternal pelvis is not remediable and but is fortunately uncommon. "Cephalo-pelvic disproportion" should not be used because it is conclusive and not descriptive. It is preferable to diagnosis "failure to progress in labor," which is reserved for those labors failing after adequate uterine contractions have been documented and labor fails to progress for 2 to 4 hours or fetal distress occurs.

Most cases of DLP are a result of **inadequate or abnormal labor forces.** Common remedial causes include unchanging supine position, analgesia (especially meperidine), early conduction anesthesia, inappropriate diagnosis of labor, and uterine dysfunction.

The above case suggests a woman with a prolonged active phase or a secondary arrest of labor. Her clinical pelvimetry and abdominal exam give no indication of fetal or pelvic abnormality. She had meperidine about 2 hours ago and contractions are beginning to become stronger again as the meperidine wears off. Mrs. Jones has not been out of bed or her supine position for the past 3 hours.

If ambulation, cessation of meperidine use, and hydration are not sufficient, augmentation of labor may be appropriate.

Augmentation of Labor

Indications for augmentation include:

- reasonable assurance that the fetus is mature
- identified fetal or maternal need for delivery
- true labor with cervical dilatation of less than 1 centimeter per hour over 2 hours

Artificial rupture of membranes will allow internal electronic monitoring of fetal heart rate and uterine contractions if appropriate and may facilitate augmentation.

Relative contraindications for augmentation are:

- false labor
- prolonged latent phase or "adequate" spontaneous contractions

- evidence of mechanical obstruction to safe delivery
- abnormal fetal presentation or uterine overdistention
- parity greater than 5 or previous uterine scar
- evidence of intrauterine fetal compromise
- inability to adequately monitor oxytocin infusion, the fetus, or contractions

Labor should be augmented only after a thorough examination of both the mother and fetus and the methods of augmentation have been discussed with the woman and her family. The indications for augmentation must be documented in the chart. When augmentation (or induction) is begun, a physician who can perform a cesarean delivery must be readily available and should be notified when the augmentation is begun. Just before initiation of the oxytocin infusion a cervical examination should be performed by the physician or the responsible person who will be monitoring the induction. The exam will assure that fetal presentation is indeed vertex, the head is well applied to the cervix, no umbilical cord can be felt, and that the current station of the fetal head and dilation and effacement of the cervix are recorded.

If the physician cannot be at the bedside or even in the labor area during the entire augmentation, a nurse who is familiar with the effects of oxytocin and who is able to identify both maternal and fetal complications must be in attendance for the woman during the entire augmentation. Uterine contraction and fetal heart rate monitoring should be done every 15 minutes. The oxytocin should be infused through a continuous volumetric pump. The physician must be immediately available to the nurse supervising the augmentation. Although this one-on-one nursing requirement may be difficult for small hospitals, oxytocin augmentation or induction requires this close evaluation.

Procedure for Augmentation of Labor

The oxytocin is administered through a peripheral intravenous line that is begun using lactated Ringer's solution. External or internal fetal electronic monitoring is useful because it allows the woman more freedom of movement and provides a permanent record of the fetus during augmentation. In addition to fetal monitoring, maternal blood pressure, pulse, and urine output should be recorded; an indwelling catheter is not appropriate in the usual case.

Whenever possible the woman should be in the lateral recumbent position except during examinations or other manipulations. Augmentation can continue with the woman in bed or positioned in a large comfortable recliner. Either will allow immediate access to the infusion pump, and will permit fetal monitoring and pelvic examination.

The starting dosage of oxytocin is 1 to 2 milliunits per minute and can be increased every 30 to 45 minutes. Some protocols call for a more rapid increase initially but this practice may be inappropriate for augmentation when the uterine reaction to the oxytocin may be more vigorous than in induction of labor. The goal of augmentation is to provide good quality contractions lasting about 60 seconds and occurring at intervals of 3 to 5 minutes. Internal uterine monitoring can be helpful when the quality of the contractions is in doubt. A deflection of 50 mm Hg pressure is consider an adequate contraction.

Although the nurse in attendance should have a protocol that allows increasing the oxytocin on a regular schedule, no verbal or telephone orders should be accepted that increase the concentration of the oxytocin in the infusion. Oxytocin should never be added to a partially filled bag of intravenous fluid, because it is impossible to ascertain the exact amount of fluid left in any bag and therefore the concentration of the oxytocin will be unknown.

Oxytocin augmentation should be stopped if contractions are more frequent than every 3 minutes; contractions last more than 60 seconds; fetal heart rate decelerations develop, especially if these are severe variable decelerations or late decelerations; or if any significant vaginal bleeding occurs.

For tetanic contractions that are not corrected by the immediate discontinuation of oxytocin, 0.25 mg of the parenteral type terbutaline can be given *subcutaneously* to produce uterine relaxation.

Documentation of oxytocin levels should not be recorded in drops or milliliters per minute but in milliunits per minute. A dose conversion chart (Table 2.2) is helpful in making this conversion.

Table 2.2 Oxytocin Dosing Chart

I. OXYTOCIN 20 UNITS PER LITER OF IV FLUID		II. OXYTOCIN 30 UNITS PER LITER OF IV FLUID	
IV Rate cc/hour	*Dose delivered milliunits/min*	*IV Rate cc/hour*	*Dose delivered Milliunits/min*
3	1	4	2
6	2	8	4
9	3	12	6
12	4	16	8
15	5	20	10
18	6	24	12
21	7	28	14
24	8	32	16
27	9	36	18
30	10	40	20

Fetal Distress

Case Report

Mandy is an 18-year-old gravida 1, para 0 woman admitted at 37 weeks gestation. She has had 10 hours of contractions, stronger and more painful in the past 2 hours. The prenatal course has been medically uneventful, but she has had problems with schoolwork and her boyfriend who has abandoned her. Her parents (your close friends) are supportive but continue to be angry and hurt. Mandy is frightened and crying. Physical exam is normal with a blood pressure of 130/82, fetal heart rate of 136 heard in the right lower quadrant, the cervix is 6 centimeters dilated, 0.5 centimeters long, and the head is at station 0 to +1. The baby is active. After a short period of observation you order a narcotic for Mandy, who rapidly becomes more calm and comfortable.

During the next hour the nurse listens through a contraction at least every 15 minutes and believes she hears decelerations of the fetal heart beat during a contraction. She is unsure whether or not they last beyond the end of the contraction. She continues listening with most contractions and applies an external tocodynamometer and a Doppler unit to monitor contractions and the fetal heart rate.

The membranes rupture spontaneously and the fluid is clear. You are able to apply a scalp electrode to confirm the pattern of variable decelerations.

Diagnosis and Treatment

Is there significant fetal distress in this case? As you observe the patient, variable decelerations continue despite the administration of oxygen by mask and turning the patient onto her side. The variable decelerations continue every 10 to 15 minutes and labor progresses rapidly. As the cervix becomes completely dilated and the patient pushes, the decelerations become more pronounced but always return to the baseline. Fetal scalp stimulation between contractions results in acceleration of the fetal heart rate by 10 to 15 beats per minute. Within 20 minutes an infant is delivered and the nuchal cord must be cut before the anterior shoulder can be delivered. The Apgar scores are 5, 7, and 9 at 1, 5, and 10 minutes; the cord pH is 7.34.

Although significant fetal distress was present in this case, this was not a severely distressed infant. The reactive scalp stimulation test, the cord pH, and the Apgar scores are reassuring.

Discussion

Normal uterine contractions restrict or even block blood flow to the placenta temporarily. The addition of umbilical cord compression with contractions can produce ominous clinical signs that may warn of hazards for the fetus even in the lowest risk pregnancy. The response of the fetus to contractions and potential hypoxic insult is assessed by fetal heart rate monitoring: the response of the heart rate to contractions and the rate of the fetal heart rate between contractions.

Recurrent late decelerations with uterine contractions (more than one or two, which disappear with position change) imply fetal compromise and can never be ignored. Variable decelerations reflect umbilical cord compression and require interventions to relieve cord compression. Variable decelerations with a slow recovery phase or a late component change this usually benign pattern into a non-reassuring pattern requiring further assessment. Fetal tachycardia (more than 160-180 beats per minute) with either variable or late decelerations may represent chronic fetal distress. Persistent fetal bradycardia (less than 100 beats per minute) is an ominous sign requiring immediate assessment and timely intervention.

Baseline heart rate has a natural variability. The accurate assessment of heart rate variability requires placement of a scalp electrode. Most decreases in fetal heart rate (FHR) variability are due to drugs given to the mother (narcotics, barbiturates, and tranquilizers) or to episodes of fetal sleep. Decreased FHR variability seen in the presence of late or marked variable decelerations should be considered a sign of fetal distress and further assessed.

When abnormalities of the FHR occur, further assessment and intervention are necessary. Immediate interventions that become part of the assessment process include:

- placing the mother in the left lateral position to decrease compression of maternal blood supply
- delivery of oxygen by mask to the mother
- gently shaking the fetus to arouse it
- discontinuing oxytocin if it is being used
- correction of hypotension from drugs or dehydration

If none of these are successful further evaluation and intervention will depend on the pattern seen and the progress of the woman in labor. If delivery is imminent (less than 15 to 30 minutes) preparations will include primarily those necessary for the infant in the delivery room such as having at least one additional experienced person available for care of the infant and reassessment of infant resuscitation equipment. If delivery will require longer than 30 minutes, further intervention will depend on the pattern seen on the FHR monitor.

Variable decelerations often disappear with changes in the mother's position, hydration of the mother, or discontinuation of analgesics or sedatives. When these maneuvers fail in the woman who has ruptured membranes and who has experienced large amounts of amniotic fluid loss, saline amnio-infusion may prove useful. This can be particularly useful to the physician who has an out-of-town consultant for cesarean sections or is having difficulty locating his or her usual obstetrics consultant.

Candidates for saline amnio-infusion are women in the first stage of labor with more than four variable decelerations not responsive to mask oxygen or position change; no ominous signs such as flat baseline, late decelerations, tachycardia, or thick meconium; and a vertex presentation with station at least 0.

Preliminary evaluation must include assessment for possible cord prolapse, dilation of the cervix, fetal presentation and station, and presence or absence of meconium in the amniotic fluid.

Preparation of the woman includes left lateral positioning with oxygen administered by mask, the placement of an intrauterine pressure catheter (IUPC) that is correctly functioning, and warming of a liter of sterile normal saline to room temperature. The bag of saline is placed 3 to 4 feet above the level of the IUPC and can be run through a blood warmer and infusion pump for warming and correct flow rate. Saline is infused at 20 milliliters per minute; the infusion is continued until decelerations stop or 500 milliliters of fluid have been given through the IUPC. If decelerations have stopped, give another 250 milliliters. Maximum fluid load is 750 to 800 milliliters. The procedure can be repeated if decelerations reoccur with repetitive fluid leakage. IUP readings may be elevated during the infusion. The infusion can be temporarily stopped to get an accurate reading.

When signs of **persistent FHR abnormalities** or fetal hypoxia persist despite simple interventions such as position changes, maternal oxygen administration, and discontinuation of oxytocin, direct assessment of the fetal acid-base status can be helpful in determining the necessity of rapid intervention. Two methods of acid-base evaluation are available: digital stimulation of the fetal scalp and fetal scalp blood sampling.

The **digital stimulation test** requires only direct access to the fetal scalp and fetal heart rate monitoring through a fetal scalp electrode. Between contractions the fetal scalp is rubbed firmly for 5 seconds. A positive and reassuring response is a 10-beat-per-minute increase in the FHR lasting at least 10 seconds. This test is considered to have few false positives, meaning that an increase in the fetal heart rate is not going to occur with a hypoxic-acidotic infant. However, a negative test does not mean that the infant is in severe distress. When the digital stimulation test is negative, fetal scalp blood sampling can further delineate the problem.

Table 2.3 Indications for Scalp Blood Sampling

Unexplained absent short-term fetal heart rate variability
Persistent late decelerations
Persistent variable decelerations with slow recovery phase (mixed deceleration
    patterns)
Unexplained persistent tachycardia
Contradicting patterns such as absent baseline variability with accelerations
Persistent bradycardia (< 100 beats per minute)
A negative fetal scalp stimulation test

Fetal scalp blood sampling requires the immediate access to blood gas testing equipment. The indications are listed in Table 2.3. The procedure begins by informing the woman and her family as fully as possible regarding the concerns about the baby and the labor. She is positioned in the left lateral position. **Supine positioning can lead to erroneous results from temporary maternal hypotension and should be avoided.** The perineum is prepped with an antiseptic solution of your choice. The endoscope is inserted into the vagina with light source attached and the fetal head is visualized and cleansed with antiseptic swabs.

Sampling takes places over one of the parietal bones; areas of edema, sutures, or fontanelle are avoided. Do not apply pressure to the endoscope because this may induce local stasis and a false reading. A thin layer of silicone lubricant is placed on the area to be sampled to promote bleeding and to retain the blood in a small area. After the fetal scalp is punctured with a lancet the blood drop is allowed to form and picked up with the end of a capillary tube. The tube is sent immediately for analysis. It is best to leave the endoscope in place until the result is known to make sure that the sample is adequate and consistent with your clinical findings.

After the amnioscope is removed, apply pressure to the area and make sure hemostasis is achieved through at least one contraction. Check periodically over the next few contractions.

Normal fetal scalp blood pH is greater than 7.24 and is reassuring. You should be able to continue observation and maternal treatment of any problems. If the fetal heart rate abnormalities persist you should repeat the sampling in 30 to 45 minutes. If the heart rate pattern deteriorates it is necessary to sample again in less than 30 minutes or take definitive action, that is, cesarean section.

Borderline pH is 7.20 to 7.24. Action will take into consideration the maternal acid-base status and the probable cause of maternal acidosis if present, the stage of labor, and clinical circumstance.

A fetal scalp blood pH less than 7.20 is abnormal. This warrants consultation and preparation for delivery as quickly as feasible.

Fortunately, complications of fetal scalp pH sampling are unusual; they include fetal bleeding and infection at the site of sampling. Careful observation after sampling should prevent the former and the latter is unlikely to be more than a superficial skin infection that will be easily treated post partum.

Contraindications for fetal scalp blood sampling are maternal bleeding disorder or a family history of hemophilia, and maternal infection with herpes, gonorrhea, and Group B streptococcus. Maternal infection with the human immunodeficiency virus and maternal carriage of hepatitis B are absolute contraindications for fetal scalp blood sampling. Any unknown fetal presentation and especially face presentations are also contraindications.

Any infant delivered operatively for fetal distress or assessed during labor for fetal distress should have (whenever available) a cord blood pH to estimate the severity of the fetal distress and to guide further resuscitation efforts of the infant.

Shoulder Dystocia

Case Report

Mrs. Anderson is in the delivery room. She is 33 years old, gravida 3, para 2, aborta 0, and has been pushing for 45 minutes and the head is crowning. The history shows a normal prenatal course, and labor has been uncomplicated and has progressed normally for a multiparous woman. You estimate the baby to be about the size of the last two, which weighed 2,700 to 2,800 grams.

Mrs. Anderson is your partner's wife and your son's favorite teacher. Her husband is in the delivery room and ready to cut the cord.

As the head emerges, you notice that it seems to come more slowly than usual and as you try to check for a nuchal cord the head slips back into the vagina between contractions. Gently directing the occiput anterior presenting head downward does nothing with the next contractions. *Your* heart rate begins to show accelerations.

Diagnosis and Treatment

Your immediate concern is shoulder dystocia. With the next contraction the head again crowns but quickly retreats into the vagina. Pulling Mrs. Anderson's thighs against her abdomen is not helpful. You explain to the Andersons that the baby's shoulders are a little large and that you will have to rotate the baby. The nurse listens to the fetal heart tones with the Doppler, reassuring everyone that the heart rate is stable and about 100 to 110 beats per minute. After cutting a medial lateral episiotomy you are able to rotate the anterior shoulder away from the symphysis and the baby delivers with the next contraction. As it cries lustily its heart rate increases to 140 beats per minute, and your heart rate falls below 100 beats per minute.

This was a moderate to severe shoulder dystocia managed by a physician who kept the family informed during her progression through procedures designed to dislodge the anterior shoulder from behind the pubic symphysis.

Discussion

Predicting or preventing shoulder dystocia is preferable to handling the situation in the delivery room. Careful identification and management of diabetes during pregnancy has greatly reduced the incidence of this problem. Risk factors for shoulder dystocia include:

- fetal weight greater than 4,000 grams or history of other babies over 4,000 grams
- maternal obesity (prepregnancy weight more than 200 pounds) or diabetes
- prolonged gestation (more than 42 weeks)
- an abnormal labor pattern, defined as arrest of dilation or prolonged second stage over 2 hours

Maternal and infant morbidity are high in shoulder dystocia. Maternal complications include hemorrhage, soft tissue damage, and, rarely, uterine rupture. Fetal mortality has been reported to be as high as 30% but is rare in modern delivery rooms. Morbidity includes brachial plexus injury and fracture of the humerus or clavicle.

Whenever possible you should have a second physician called immediately to assist with the delivery and the infant. **Remember that because the shoulder dystocia results from entrapment of the anterior shoulder behind the symphysis pubis, downward traction on the fetal head and neck are not going to facilitate delivery and may damage the infant.**

An initial maneuver is to have an assistant apply suprapubic pressure while you try to rotate the fetal shoulder from under the public symphysis to under the pubic ramus. This may be accomplished with or without a contraction and both should be tried.

If this fails, flex the maternal hips and push the thighs against the maternal abdomen. This changes the direction of the contraction forces and often allows the shoulders to be rotated or slipped under the symphysis. Do not rotate the hips too far to the side. Repeat the suprapubic pressure if necessary.

If the first two maneuvers fail, extend the episiotomy (into the rectum if necessary) and attempt delivery of the posterior arm. Insert your hand along the posterior wall of the vagina and along the sacral curve. Find the infant's posterior arm and sweep the forearm across the chest and face and out the introitus. If you can not tell which direction is "across the chest" reach into the antecubital fossa and identify the elbow. Do not use the axilla as a pressure point because this may cause nerve injury. You now have an infant with the posterior arm extending beyond the head. The bi-shoulder diameter has been reduced and the infant may be deliverable.

If you still cannot deliver the anterior shoulder you can attempt the Wood's maneuver. Rotate the posterior shoulder 180 degrees in the direction of the baby's back with an assistant applying fundal pressure so that the anterior shoulder will end up below the symphysis pubis.

In rare cases the infant's clavicle may have to be fractured to accomplish delivery. If recognized immediately and explained to the parents, clavicle fractures rarely require specific treatment or cause any permanent disability or disfigurement.

If all maneuvers fail the head should be rotated to the occiput posterior position, flexed, and reintroduced into the maternal pelvis. An emergency cesarean section will be necessary. Tocolysis with intravenous or subcutaneous ritodrine or terbutaline can be helpful and may decrease cord compression during contractions.

Unique Rural Situations

In rural areas access to consultants and tertiary care centers can be limited by problems of time, distance, weather, and cultural norms. Practices that may seem strange to an urban family physician are appropriate and necessary in rural areas. It is good medical practice to have a woman at term with a history of precipitous delivery come to stay in town or even at the hospital as the blizzard or the torrential rains approach.

The appropriate time to transfer to a tertiary care center a woman with preterm labor you have been able to stop quickly may have to vary depending on road and weather conditions. Helicopter transport is widely available, but helicopters cannot fly in dense fog, blizzards, sand storms, and electrical storms. Some mountain villages are not accessible by any aircraft. The rural physician will have to refer with greater care and forethought than the urban physician who finds help down the hall or down the street.

Recommended Reading

Clark, S. L., Phelan, J. P., & Corton, D. B. (1988). *Critical care obstetrics.* Oradell, NJ: Medical Economics Books.

Queenan, J. T. (Ed.). (1986). *Management of high risk pregnancy* (2nd ed.). Oradell, NJ: Medical Economics Books.

Queenan, J. T., & Hobbins, J. C. (Eds.). (1987). *Procotols for high risk pregnancies* (2nd ed.). Oradell, NJ: Medical Economics Books.

3
■ ■ ■

Stabilization and Transport
of the Ill Newborn Infant

THEODORE R. THOMPSON

Introduction

Transport of the high-risk pregnant woman and her fetus or the ill newborn infant to a neonatal intensive care unit (NICU) requires a safe, coordinated, and organized system. The majority of high-risk pregnant women can be identified before delivery. The safest, most comfortable, warmest, quietest, least expensive, and most efficient mode of neonatal transport is maternal transport with the fetus in utero. However, about one third of newborn infants requiring intensive care are born to mothers presenting too late in preterm labor or too ill to be safely transported, have anomalies first noted after birth, or develop problems after delivery. This chapter addresses the appropriate steps in the resuscitation and stabilization of these infants while awaiting the arrival of neonatal transport personnel from the referral newborn intensive care unit.

Resuscitation

Approximately two thirds of newborn infants requiring delivery room assistance can be anticipated before delivery. Table 3.1 outlines high-risk maternal conditions that may be associated with the delivery of a depressed infant. The remaining one third of infants needing assistance in the delivery room cannot be identified before delivery; thus, someone skilled in resuscitation should always be present to attend to the infant.

Table 3.1 High-Risk Maternal and Fetal Conditions That May Be Associated With Delivery of a Depressed Infant

---

A. Maternal Factors

1. Maternal disease including diabetes mellitus, hypertension, renal disease, cardiac disease, drug addiction, alcoholism, disorder or trauma requiring surgery.
2. Premature labor or premature rupture of membranes. The smaller the infant, the greater the likelihood that the infant will be depressed at birth.
3. Pregnancy-induced hypertension (preeclampsia).
4. Multiple gestation.
5. Prolonged gestation (above 42 weeks).
6. Prolonged rupture of membranes (more than 18-24 hours).
7. Severe isoimmunization (Rh or other blood group antigen).
8. Polyhydramnios, oligohydramnios.
9. Lack of prenatal care.
10. Previous antenatal, perinatal, neonatal death(s).

B. Labor and Delivery Factors

1. Placental accident-hemorrhage, including:
    a. Abruptio placenta
    b. Placenta praevia
2. Cesarean section (high-risk maternal factors)
3. Abnormal presentation (breech, transverse, face, brow)
4. Fetal distress
    a. Fetal heart tones persistently more than 160 or less than 120/minute
    b. Loss of baseline variability in absence of depressant drugs
    c. Fetal acidosis (pH < 7.10-7.15)
    d. Severe variable or late decelerations, or sinusoidal patterns on fetal monitoring
    e. Thick, meconium-stained amniotic fluid; absent fetal heart rate accelerations and/or presence of tachycardia (oligohydramnios may be present)
5. Prolapsed, knotted, compressed cord
6. Prolonged or obstructed labor: prolonged second stage of labor
7. Maternal fever, hypotension
8. Depressant drugs given to mother near delivery

C. Fetal factors

1. Anomalies (e.g., diaphragmatic hernia)
2. Hydrops
3. Intrauterine growth retardation

The temperature of the delivery room area must be kept above 70°-72°F to reduce the risk of hypothermia. Placing the newborn infant in a radiant warmer to provide a neutral thermal environment and drying the infant, including the scalp, will reduce morbidity. The scalp should be covered after drying and wet linens and blankets should be replaced to further reduce heat loss. Gentle bulb suctioning with the head slightly down and gentle tactile stimulation are then performed.

Immediate evaluation of the infant in the delivery room and subsequent decision making about medical care involves three clinical parameters:

- respiratory effort
- heart rate
- color

Although Apgar scores should be recorded at 1 and 5 minutes after birth, waiting for 1 minute to evaluate the infant only delays initiating appropriate resuscitative efforts. Use of a mnemonic will facilitate resuscitation:

- Anticipation—High-risk woman or fetus
- Recognition—Respiratory effort
     Heart rate
     Color
- Correction
     A: Airway
     B: Breathing
     C: Circulation—cardiac massage
     D: Drugs—Epinephrine, colloid, NaHCO$_3$, naloxone, glucose
     E: Environment—neutral thermal environment

More than 95% of infants will respond to establishment of an adequate airway and initiation of breathing with positive pressure ventilation and 100% oxygen while maintaining a neutral thermal environment. Indications for positive pressure ventilation at a rate of 40-60 breaths per minute with 100% oxygen include:

36   EXPLORING RURAL MEDICINE

Table 3.2 Endotracheal Intubation of Newborn Infants

Birth Weight (grams)/ Gestational Age (weeks)	Internal Diameter (mm)*	End Tip of ET Tube to Lower Lip Distance (cm) (number at lower lip)**
Below 1,000/27	2.5	6-7
1,000/27-28	2.5-3.0	7
2,000/32-34	3.0-3.5	8
3,000/37-40	3.5-4.0	9
4,000/Above 39 Weeks	4.0	10

NOTES: *Most useful straight ET tube: 3.0 mm internal diameter (3.5-4.0 mm for full term), 13 cm length
**Cut at least 1.0-1.5 cm longer

- apnea
- gasping respiratory efforts
- a heart rate below 100 beats per minute

Many infants below 31 weeks gestation (1,500 grams) require ventilatory assistance in the delivery room. A face mask of the appropriate size and an infant resuscitation bag, with oxygen reservoir for self-inflating bags, are necessary to provide effective ventilation. Familiarity with the type of infant bag used at your hospital is essential; some have inspiratory pressure limits of 35-40 cm of water whereas others do not. The technique of mask and bag ventilation requires practice. When performing mask and bag ventilation, ensure that the airway is clear and that an orogastric tube is in place (left open to atmospheric pressure). Slightly hyperextend the neck and lift the jaw while keeping the fingers away from below the chin area. Observe the infant for return of heart rate and color, bilateral chest expansion, and equal bilateral breath sounds on auscultation.

Bagging via an appropriate sized endotracheal (ET) tube (Table 3.2) rather than the mask provides for delivery of increased tidal volume. Positive pressure ventilation should begin at a rate of 40-60 breaths per minute, a pressure of 30-40 cm of water, and 100% oxygen. The pressure can often be decreased to 20-40 cm of water after the initial several breaths. Once inserted, the ET tube needs to be securely taped in place and a chest X ray should be obtained to check for positioning of the tip of the tube.

Chest compressions (cardiac massage) should be initiated for the infant whose heart rate remains below 60 or between 60 and 80 beats per minute and is not increasing after positive pressure ventilation with 100% oxygen for 15-30 seconds. The two-finger technique or application of both thumbs to the lower one third of the sternum, with fingers wrapped around the vertebral column, is recommended at a rate of about 120 beats per minute. Using a ratio of breathing to compressions and interruption of compressions for breathing are not currently recommended for the neonate.

Drugs are rarely necessary for the resuscitation of the neonate, but appropriate medications should be available (Figure 3.1). Glucose may be needed because many infants who are depressed at birth have depleted glycogen stores. Epinephrine and naloxone can be given via the endotracheal tube or intravenously. Other medications should be given intravenously via a 3.5 or 5 French end-hole catheter inserted into the umbilical vein until blood returns (usually 3-4 cm).

Consideration of Transfer of the Infant to an NICU

Any resuscitation beyond minimal bagging and low flow oxygen should initiate the consideration of transfer of the newborn infant to a neonatal intensive care unit. Indications for transport of the ill newborn infant to an NICU vary, depending on the skill and experience of the physician and staff providing 24-hour care to the infant and the availability of appropriate equipment and ancillary services. Tables 3.3 and 3.4 feature neonatal complications and high-risk situations that are common reasons for consultation and neonatal transport. The decision for transport should always be made jointly by referring and consulting physicians. For most infants requiring special care, neonatologists agree that transport can usually be better accomplished by dispatching the specially trained and skilled team from the NICU to the infant at the referring facility. Intensive care therapy can then be initiated at the referring hospital and maintained during transport. For infants who are very stable, transfer utilizing personnel from the referring hospital may be considered after appropriate discussion.

text continues on p. 40

Drug or Volume Expander and Indication	Concentration to Administer	Preparation (based on recommended concentration)	Dosage and Route	Rate and Precautions
Epinephrine Heart rate of zero or below 80 despite IPPV and 100% oxygen for 30 seconds	1:10,000	1 ml in a syringe Can dilute 1:1 with normal saline if giving ET	0.1-0.3 ml/kg IV or ET	Give rapidly
Volume Expanders Evidence of hypovolemia	Whole blood 5% albumin Plasma protein fraction Normal saline Ringer's Lactate	40 ml given by syringe or IV drip	10 ml/kg IV	Give over 5-10 min
Sodium Bicarbonate Documented or assumed acidosis	0.5 mEq/ml (4.2% solution)	20 ml in a syringe or two 10 ml prefilled syringes	2 mEq/kg IV	Give slowly at least 2 min and only after effective oxygenation
Naloxone Hydrochloride Respiratory depression with maternal narcotic administration	Adult Narcan 1.0 mg/ml 0.4 mg/ml	1 ml in a syringe Can dilute 1:1 with normal saline if giving ET	0.1 mg/kg (0.1 ml/kg for 1.0 mg/ml solution) (0.25 ml/kg for 0.4 mg/ml solution)	Give rapidly only after effective oxygenation; may need to repeat
Glucose Restore glucose levels	10% solution	20 ml in syringe	2 ml/kg bolus then 72-96 ml/kg/day IV	Continuous infusion

Figure 3.1. Medications for Resuscitation of Newborn Infants

Table 3.3 Potential High-Risk Neonatal Conditions

A. Perinatal Distress

    1. Prolonged hypotonia and/or poor respiratory effort

    2. Combined 1- and 5-minute Apgar scores < 6, which may be associated with:

        a. Central nervous system—seizures, cerebral edema

        b. Pulmonary—meconium aspiration, respiratory distress syndrome, "shock" lung, hemorrhage

        c. Cardiac—congestive heart failure

        d. Renal—acute renal failure

        e. Gastrointestinal—ulcer, vomiting, necrotizing enterocolitis

        f. Hematological—disseminated intravascular coagulopathy, thrombocytopenia

    3. Meconium staining, fetal distress with intrauterine growth retardation

B. Respiratory Distress (RDS score > 4)

    1. Persistent tachypnea > 60-80 breaths/minute

    2. Grunting

    3. Retractions

    4. Cyanosis in room air

    5. Decreased air entry

    6. Apneic episodes

    7. Flaring nares

    8. Stridor, wheezing

C. Cyanosis (central)

    1. Pulmonary disorders: medical/surgical cause, pulmonary hypertension

    2. Congenital heart disease (often not responsive to 100% oxygen)

    3. Metabolic (e.g., hypoglycemia, hypocalcemia)

    4. Central nervous system disorder

    5. Shock

    6. Sepsis

    7. Hematologic abnormality (e.g., methemoglobinemia)

E. Prematurity: < 37 weeks' gestation

F. Post-term: > 42 weeks' gestation

G. Small or large for gestational age (SGA, LGA)

H. Infant of a diabetic mother (often LGA)

I. Central nervous signs, symptoms: seizures, tremors, irritability, jitteriness, lethargy, hypertonia, hypotonia

(Continued)

Table 3.3 (Continued)

J. Gastrointestinal signs, symptoms: abdominal distention, persistent poor feeding, vomiting (particularly bilious), delayed stooling (> 24 hours)

K. Delayed voiding (> 24 hours)

L. Congenital malformation involving central nervous system, genitourinary, gastrointestinal, pulmonary and/or cardiovascular systems, often requiring surgery

M. Jaundice (total bilirubin > 5 mg% in first 24 hours, any indirect bilirubin > 12-18 mg/dl, dependent on gestational age and postnatal age; Rh sensitization with hyperbilirubinemia; and/or elevated direct bilirubin)

N. Thermal instability (hypo- and hyperthermia)

O. Hypotension, poor perfusion, evidence of blood loss

P. Anemia; thrombocytopenia-petechiae; hemorrhagic diathesis; polycythemia (umbilical venous hematocrit > 65%, peripheral venous hematocrit > 63%)

Q. Skin lesions suggestive of infection

R. Infection

S. "Not looking right"; "not acting right"

Stabilization

Once the infant has been successfully resuscitated, attention must be directed to stabilization procedures to reduce morbidity and mortality and to improve the efficiency of transport. Stabilization of any infant involves anticipating and preventing or rapidly detecting and correcting the five Hs plus acidosis (Table 3.5).

In addition, most ill newborn infants require vascular access for administration of fluids, emergency infusion of drugs, monitoring of arterial blood gases, and perhaps monitoring of blood pressure. Placement of peripheral intravenous lines is often difficult in the newborn infant. Many authorities recommend the placement of umbilical venous and/or umbilical artery catheters for immediate vascular access. For the umbilical artery catheter (UAC), a 3.5 or 5 French end-hole catheter can be inserted into one of the two arteries.

Table 3.4 Suggested Reasons for Considering Consultation and Possible Transport of the Newborn Infant

1. Respiratory distress
   a. Downes or RDS score > 4-5
   b. Arterial oxygen tension (PaO_2) < 60 torr in FIO2 0.4-0.5
   c. Requirement of FIO2 > 0.4 to relieve cyanosis
   d. Arterial carbon dioxide tension ($PaCO_2$) > 55 torr or rapidly rising $PaCO_2$ (> 5-10 torr/hour)
   e. Arterial pH persistently < 7.25
   f. Apneic episodes
   g. Limited capacity to monitor inspired oxygen concentration, arterial blood gases
   h. Limited capacity to administer precise intravenous fluid infusion

2. Surgical emergencies including
   a. Pneumothorax
   b. Intestinal obstruction (e.g., atresia, malrotation- volvulus, Hirschsprung's)
   c. Omphalocele/gastroschisis
   d. Neural tube defect (e.g., myelomeningocele)
   e. Abdominal mass
   f. Diaphragmatic hernia
   g. Esophageal atresia with or without distal tracheoesophageal fistula
   h. Choanal atresia

3. Suspected congenital heart disease

4. Birth weight < 1,500 grams and/or gestational age < 31-32 weeks

5. Severe perinatal distress (particularly with persistent hypotonia, seizures, and/or when the combined 1- and 5-minute Apgar scores are < 6)

6. Infection (bacterial, viral)

7. "Not doing well" for an unknown reason

Table 3.5 The Five H's Plus Acidosis

Abnormality	Prevention or Correction
Hypothermia	Neutral thermal environment
Hypotension	Colloid infusion; inotropic agents
Hypoglycemia	Infusion of glucose solution (10%)
Hypoxemia	Oxygen administration
Hypercapnia	Alveolar ventilation
Acidosis	Metabolic colloid
	Respiratory alveolar ventilation

Placement of its tip between vertebral bodies T6-T9 can usually be accomplished by inserting the catheter about one third of the infant's crown-to-heel length. The tip of the UAC should not be kept between bodies T1-T3 because major arterial branches diverge from the aorta in this region. Many neonatologists prefer to lower the UAC tip to vertebral bodies L3-L4. Normal saline with 0.5 units of heparin per milliliter is usually infused by pump at 1 ml/hour into the UAC; glucose solutions may be infused at more rapid rates with lower heparin concentrations. For the umbilical venous catheter (UVC), a 3.5 or 5 French end-hole catheter can be inserted on a temporary basis into the large, patulous umbilical vein until blood returns, usually 3-4 centimeters, for infusion of glucose solutions, colloid, and emergency drugs. If the UVC is to remain for a long time, the catheter tip should be situated at the entrance of the inferior vena cava into the right atrium, which is accomplished by inserting the catheter one half of the distance used for the umbilical artery catheter tip placement at T6-T9 plus one centimeter. Glucose solutions can be administered through the UVC using an infusion pump at a rate of 3-4 ml/kg/hr (72-96 ml/kg/day).

Hypothermia

Hypothermia increases the metabolic rate and oxygen consumption for newborn infants, and thus may potentiate hypotension, hypoglycemia, apnea, metabolic acidosis, and hypoxemia. This cascade may result in reversion to fetal circulation secondary to an increase in pulmonary vascular resistance. Hypothermia occurs most frequently in those infants who are least able to tolerate stress: the premature infant, with the risk of hypothermia increasing as gestational age and birth weight decrease; the infant who requires resuscitative efforts at birth; and the infant who requires supplemental oxygen.

Prevention of hypothermia begins in the delivery room. Heat loss can be reduced by placing the infant in a radiant warmer and by drying of the skin and scalp. If a warmer is not available, a prewarmed isolette or prewarmed blankets can be used. The most effective method to maintain a neutral thermal environment for the infant is to utilize Servo control on the warmer or isolette to maintain the infant's skin temperature at 97°-98°F. Axillary temperatures should be checked until stable at 97°-98°F. A rectal temperature should be checked only if axillary temperatures remain low. To minimize the risk of intestinal perforation when checking the rectal temperature, care must be exercised to ensure that the lubricated thermometer is not inserted too far.

The infant who is hypothermic can be rewarmed with commercial warmers covered by warm blankets. Rewarming should be undertaken at approximately one degree per hour, until the normal axillary temperature of 97°-98°F is reached. Normal rectal temperature is 98°-98.6°F.

Hypotension

Hypotension is common in ill newborn infants. Infants at greatest risk for hypoperfusion with low blood pressure include those with the following conditions:

- mothers with vaginal bleeding within 3 weeks of delivery, particularly if due to placental abruption or placenta praevia
- infection, especially due to group B streptococci
- respiratory distress
- perinatal distress associated with decreased myocardial function
- intestinal obstruction, gastroschisis or omphalocele
- congenital heart disease

Clinical signs and symptoms of hypotension include:

- capillary refill greater than 4 seconds
- decreased peripheral pulses with a good heart rate
- cool, mottled distal extremities
- pallor despite good oxygenation

The blood pressure of a newborn infant can be monitored peripherally with various noninvasive blood pressure monitors. Central blood pressure monitoring can be done with an umbilical artery or radial artery catheter attached to a transducer. The correlation between noninvasive and direct intra-arterial blood pressure monitoring is good, except the noninvasive method may overestimate blood pressures in hypotensive infants. Most preterm infants have a systolic blood pressure greater than 40 torr, with a mean greater than 25-30 torr. Full-term infants usually have systolic blood pressures above 50 torr, with a mean greater than 40 torr. A useful rule of thumb is that the lowest acceptable mean blood pressure is equal to the gestational age in weeks of the infant. Hypotension is managed by the following methods:

1. Slow infusion of colloid, particularly in premature infants: 10 ml/kg IV (e.g., human plasma protein fraction, 5% albumin, fresh frozen plasma, packed red cells); may repeat once.
2. Continuous infusion (infusion pump) of an inotropic agent IV (e.g., via umbilical venous catheter): Dopamine 2.5-10 mcg/kg/min; Dobutamine 10-20 mcg/kg/min

   Infusion formula: milligrams of dopamine or dobutamine to add to 100 ml of IV fluid =

   $$\frac{\text{dose rate (mcg/kg/min)} \times \text{weight (kg)} \times 6}{\text{infusion rate (ml/hr, usually } 0.5-1.0 \text{ ml/hr)}}$$

Normal mean and systolic blood pressures are given in Table 3.6.

Hypoglycemia

Sick newborn infants rapidly exhaust their glycogen stores and are prone to develop hypoglycemia, defined as a blood glucose level less than 40 mg/dL or a serum glucose less than 45 mg/dL. Common conditions that increase the risk of neonatal hypoglycemia are:

- prematurity
- intrauterine growth retardation
- respiratory distress
- perinatal distress
- hypothermia
- infection
- lack of significant intake by 16-24 hours after birth
- maternal diabetes mellitus

Table 3.6 Normal Mean and Systolic Blood Pressures

	Systolic	Mean
Preterm	> 40	> 25–30
Term	> 50	> 40

To reduce the risk of hypoglycemia, a glucose solution such as 10% dextrose solution at 3-4 ml/kg/hr can be infused via peripheral vein, an umbilical venous catheter, or an umbilical artery catheter. Infants who have serum glucose levels below 45 mg/dL should receive glucose intravenously or orally, depending on the stability of the infant.

Hypoglycemia is managed by infusing a bolus of 10% glucose and water (2 ml/kg) followed by continuous infusion of a 10%-12% dextrose solution at 3-4 ml/kg/hr by pump. Serum or blood glucose levels are monitored and the rate is adjusted as needed. Because of their hypertonicity, 25% and 50% glucose solutions are now rarely used.

Hypoxemia

Respiratory distress is the most common indicator for admission to an NICU. Prompt attention to hypoxemia (PaO_2 < 50 torr), hypercapnia, and acidosis is extremely important to reduce morbidity and prevent mortality, and to prevent reversion to the fetal circulatory pattern. The history and physical examination of the infant with respiratory distress provide specific clinical clues to the underlying cause of the respiratory distress and appropriate evaluation and therapy (Table 3.7).

The Respiratory Distress Syndrome (RDS) or Downes score (Figure 3.2) is a clinical scoring system that can assist with decisions about further care. A score of 4 or more implies respiratory distress, and a score of 8 or more implies impending respiratory failure, often with the need to initiate positive pressure ventilation. If the infant requires long distance transport, intubation and ventilation may be indicated for a score of 6 or greater, depending on the clinical situation.

Table 3.7 Selected Clinical Information and Most Common Associated
Clinical Disorders Causing Neonatal Respiratory Distress

Clinical Information	Most Likely Disorder(s)
1. Prematurity	1. Respiratory distress syndrome (RDS); perinatal depression
2. Infant of diabetic mother	2. RDS; wet lung (transient tachypnea of the newborn); congenital heart disease; persistent pulmonary hypertension (PPH)
3. Cesarean delivery	3. Wet lung; RDS (particularly without preceding labor); perinatal depression
4. Post-term	4. Meconium aspiration; perinatal depression; "shock" lung; PPH
5. Intrauterine growth retardation	5. Meconium aspiration; perinatal depression; "shock" lung; PPH
6. Meconium-stained fluid	6. Meconium aspiration; perinatal depression; "shock" lung; PPH
7. Maternal infection (e.g., chorio-amnionitis, UTI)	7. Pneumonia
8. Polyhydramnios; excessive secretions	8. Esophageal atresia with or without distal fistula; central nervous system abnormality
9. Oligohydramnios	9. Pulmonary hypoplasia (e.g., Potter's, pneumothorax); aspiration syndrome; PPH
10. Apneic episodes	10. Pneumonia; RDS; metabolic (e.g., hypoglycemia) or central nervous system abnormality
11. Pleural effusion	11. Pneumonia; chylothorax; wet lung
12. Brachial plexus injury	12. Phrenic nerve paralysis (ipsilateral)
13. Tachypnea alone— minimal distress	13. Wet lung; congenital heart disease
14. Persistent cyanosis in FIO2 1.0	14. Cyanotic congenital heart disease; PPH
15. Right-sided heart tones	15. Diaphragmatic hernia; left pneumothorax; dextrocardia

Score	0	1	2
Cyanosis	None	In room air	In 40% O_2
Retractions	None	Mild	Severe
Grunting	None	Audible with stethoscope	Audible without stethoscope
Air entry (crying)	Clear	Decreased or delayed	Barely audible
Respiratory rate	Under 60	60–80	Over 80 or apnea

Figure 3.2. RDS or Downs Scoring System

NOTE: Clinical respiratory distress: > 4 for 2 hours during first 8 hours of life; need for blood gas monitoring. Impending respiratory failure: both ≥.

The sick newborn infant's skin color is not a reliable indicator of oxygenation. Cyanosis may not appear in newborn infants until the PaO_2 level is below 40-45 torr, when tissue perfusion may be impaired and pulmonary hypertension may develop with reversion to the fetal circulation. Arterial blood gas values provide a more objective measurement of hypoxemia. Insertion of an umbilical or peripheral artery catheter provides the capability of monitoring PaO_2 as well as pH and $PaCO_2$ levels. Venous and capillary pO_2 values are not very helpful.

Pulse oximetry to determine oxygen saturation (SAO_2) levels has become very useful in monitoring the infant's oxygenation status. Although it should not replace blood gases it is a very useful adjunct, especially in hospitals where serial performance of blood gases is difficult. Normal and abnormal newborn respiratory parameters are illustrated in Table 3.8.

Furthermore, hyperoxia cannot be detected by clinical observation. Pulse oximetry does not always permit detection of hyperoxia when values are above 96%, and does not provide information on acid-base balance.

Hypoxemia can often be prevented or corrected by the delivery of warm, humidified oxygen via headbox, a funnel, or tubing placed 0.5 inches from the nares. The oxygen flow rate should be 5 liters per minute if delivered via the funnel or tubing, or 8-10 liters per

Table 3.8 Normal and Abnormal Newborn Respiratory Parameters

	Normal	*Respiratory Failure*
pH	7.30-7.40	< 7.25
$PaCO_2$	30-35 torr	> 55-60 torr
PaO_2*	> 60 torr	< 50-60 torr
	(room air)	(FIO_2 0.4-0.5)
SaO_2	> 90-96%**	< 85%

NOTES: *For infants with lung disease, not heart disease.
            **May need SaO_2 above 96% if there is a high risk for pulmonary hypertension.

minute when delivered into a headbox. Delivery of oxygen directly into an isolette will not permit an oxygen concentration of more than 30%-40%. If a blender is available with compressed air and oxygen, a specific concentration of oxygen can be delivered. FIO2 levels should be monitored when administering oxygen.

- Normal PaO_2 = 60-80 torr
- Normal SaO_2 = 90%-96%

Hypercapnia

Hypercapnia is defined as a $PaCO_2$ value greater than 45-55 torr and is often accompanied by a pH below 7.25. Arterial blood samples provide the most accurate method to monitor $PaCO_2$ levels; capillary samples may be useful to follow trends. Infants with hypercapnia and low pH values usually need ventilatory assistance. Positive pressure ventilation is provided by a bag or ventilator with an appropriately sized, tight-fitting mask or endotracheal tube (Table 3.2) at an initial rate of 40-60 breaths per minute, peak inspiratory pressure by manometry of 20-40 centimeters of water, positive end-expiratory pressure (PEEP) of 3-5 centimeters of water, and FIO2 of 1.0. Changes in rate, peak inspiratory pressure, PEEP level, and FIO2 may be required, depending on arterial blood gas and SaO_2 values. Ventilation via an endotracheal tube provides better tidal volume delivery but is difficult and potentially dangerous for those not skilled in ET tube placement in newborns. Most situations can be handled by continuous bag and mask ventilation until the transport team arrives. The normal newborn $PaCO_2$ is 35-45 torr.

Acidosis

Metabolic and respiratory acidosis commonly develop in ill newborn infants. Metabolic acidosis occurs with hypoperfusion and inadequate oxygen delivery. With metabolic acidosis, the pH is low, the pCO_2 is normal or low, and the base deficit or negative base excess is greater than 5-6 milliequivalents per liter. A laboratory can help to compute the base deficit.

Management of **metabolic acidosis** consists of ensuring adequate tissue oxygenation and perfusion, followed by the infusion of sodium bicarbonate at a rate not to exceed 1 milliequivalent per kilogram per minute. The 0.5 mEq/L (4.2%) solution of sodium bicarbonate should be utilized. The initial amount to infuse is 2 mEq/kg or can be calculated as follows:

number of mEq of sodium bicarbonate =
(base deficit × birth weight [kg] × 0.3)/2.

Management of **respiratory acidosis** with a low pH and high PaCO2 is to increase alveolar ventilation. Sodium bicarbonate may be detrimental to such infants. The normal newborn arterial pH is 7.30-7.40.

Ventilation

Although simple bag and mask ventilation is sufficient for many babies, those with severe respiratory distress syndrome, marked prematurity, or sepsis may require positive pressure ventilation with positive end expiratory pressure (PEEP). The indications for positive pressure ventilation include:

1. Downes or RDS score ≥ 8 (consider ≥ 6 for long distance transport)
2. Severe apneic episodes, gasping respiratory efforts, pH < 7.25 AND $PaCO_2$ < 55-60 torr or rapidly rising $PaCO_2$ level (> 5-10 torr/hour)
3. Birth weight < 1,500 grams and/or gestational age < 31 weeks for many infants unless vigorous
4. Failure of nasal CPAP: PaO2 < 60 torr, FIO2 = 0.6, CPAP = 6 cm water
5. pH < 7.20 despite appropriate therapy (metabolic/respiratory acidosis)

Table 3.9 General Measures in Stabilizing the Ill Newborn Infant

A. Administer vitamin K1 oxide, 1 mg IM

B. Monitor vital signs, including Downes or RDS score

C. Insert orogastric tube for decompression; place NPO

D. Record urination, meconium passage

E. Ensure vascular access

    1. Umbilical artery and/or venous catheter, peripheral IV

        a. Infusion pump
        b. 10% glucose solution, 72-96 ml/kg/day

F. Consider administration of antibiotics after obtaining blood and other appropriate cultures

    1. Ampicillin, 100 mg/kg/day in two divided doses IV or IM and
    2. Gentamicin, 5 mg/kg/day in two divided doses IV or IM or
    3. Cefotaxime, 100 mg/kg/day in two divided doses IV

G. Cover omphalocele, gastroschisis, or myelomeningocele with sterile gauze pads moistened with sterile, warmed normal saline, and enclose in plastic covering

H. Obtain a maternal vaginal culture

I. Obtain 5-10 ml of maternal blood (clotted)

J. Provide X rays, photocopies of maternal and infant charts

K. Explain to parents why, by whom, and where their infant will be transported, and provide emotional support to parents

6. Shock or marked hypoperfusion
7. Diaphragmatic hernia
8. Ineffective ventilation via bag and mask
9. Thick meconium or blood-stained amniotic fluid
10. Severe pulmonary disease
11. Esophageal atresia with or without a distal tracheo-esophageal fistula.

General Measures

Table 3.9 outlines general supportive measures to be used in stabilizing any ill newborn infant. Communication with the parents

Table 3.10 Causes of Abnormal Chest X-Ray Findings in Newborn Infants

Common Medical Causes	Common Surgical Causes
Respiratory distress syndrome— hyaline membrane disease	Pneumothorax
Wet lung—transient tachypnea	Diaphragmatic hernia
Pneumonia	Pleural effusion
Aspiration	Esophageal atresia with or without tracheoesophageal fistula
Hemorrhage	Lobar emphysema
Pulmonary insufficiency— immaturity	Cyst
Congestive heart failure— pulmonary edema	Mass
Pulmonary hypoplasia	

and the referring physician and staff is an extremely important aspect in the delivery of quality care. The transport team can explain to the parents the basic routines of the NICU, the initial problems of the infant, and the anticipated management plan. The parents should be encouraged to touch and hold their infant, even when the infant is extremely ill. Parents should also be encouraged to visit and be with their infant on the NICU whenever possible. Finally, the physicians and nurses caring for the mother must be kept informed of the infant's problems and progress to provide adequate ongoing emotional support to the parents. Consultants and NICU personnel must never be "too busy" to provide regular updates.

Additional laboratory and X-ray evaluation is helpful and should include a chest X ray to determine if a medical or a surgical condition is responsible for the infant's respiratory distress (Table 3.10). Finally, serum glucose levels, central hematocrit, platelet count, and white blood cell count with differential are helpful. Appropriate cultures, including a blood culture, should also be obtained before starting antibiotics. A maternal vaginal culture, particularly for group B streptococci, is often useful.

Summary

The maternal uterus remains the preferred mode of transport of high-risk neonates. However, transportation of the mother is not always possible, and problems affecting the newborn infant cannot always be anticipated before delivery. Thus, skill in resuscitation and stabilization procedures is essential. Resuscitation is based on evaluation of the infant's respiratory effort, heart rate, and skin color. Management is directed toward providing an appropriate airway, breathing for the infant, and maintaining a neutral thermal environment. The care provided before the arrival of the transport team is important in reducing the morbidity and mortality for ill newborn infants and will improve their outcome.

Recommended Reading

American Academy of Pediatrics, Committee on Fetus and Newborn and American College of Obstetricians and Gynecologists, Committee on Obstetrics. (1988). *Maternal and fetal medicine. Guidelines for perinatal care* (2nd ed.). Elk Grove Village, IL: Author.

American Heart Association and American Academy of Pediatrics. (1990). *Textbook of neonatal resuscitation*. Elk Grove Village, IL: Author.

Avery, G. B. (Ed.). (1987). *Neonatology. Pathophysiology and management of the newborn* (3rd ed.). Philadelphia: J. B. Lippincott.

Downes, J. J., Vidyasagar, D., Morrow, G. M., & Boggs, T. R. (1970). Respiratory distress syndrome of newborn infants. I. New clinical scoring system (RDS score) with acid-base and blood gas correlations. *Clinical Pediatrics, 9,* 325.

Fanaroff, A. A., & Klaus, M. H. (1986). Transportation of the high-risk infant. In M. H. Klaus & A. A. Fanaroff (Eds.), *Care of the high-risk neonate* (3rd ed.) (pp. 387-395). Philadelphia: W. B. Saunders.

Pernoll, M. L., Benda, G. I., & Babson, S. G. (1986). *Diagnosis and management of the fetus and neonate at risk: A guide for team care* (5th ed.). St. Louis: C. V. Mosby.

Thompson, T. R. (Ed.) (1983). *Intensive care of newborn infants: A practical manual.* Minneapolis: University of Minnesota Press.

Thompson, T. R. (1981). Stabilization and transport of the critically ill newborn infant. In D. F. Roberts (Ed.), *Neonatal resuscitation: A practical guide.* New York: Academic Press.

4
∎ ∎ ∎

Bronchopulmonary Dysplasia:
After the Infant Goes Home

JOHN J. McNAMARA

NANCY N. HOOGENHOUS

Introduction

As teams of rural primary and urban tertiary care providers save more healthy preterm infants, they also save more damaged and disabled preterm babies. These children are surviving very complicated and prolonged postnatal courses. Some will experience other developmental delays and complications, such as retrolental fibroplasia and chronic respiratory dysfunction due to bronchopulmonary dysplasia (BPD). A few of these fragile babies will return home dependent on sophisticated life-sustaining equipment. On-site care for these children will become the responsibility of the family physician. This section will provide an outline of the complex care of babies with BPD.

What is bronchopulmonary dysplasia? Pathologically, it consists of areas of air trapping, alternating with areas of collapse, enlargement of smooth muscle bundles surrounding airways, interstitial edema, and scar formation. Clinically, BPD is characterized by chronic respiratory difficulties and persistent pulmonary changes on chest X ray. Functional impairment varies from mild tachypnea to respiratory failure requiring supplemental oxygen or mechanical ventilation. Children with BPD have both obstructive and restrictive disease, and have associated problems with nutrition, developmental delay, retrolental fibroplasia, and a high incidence of airway reactivity.

Infants with pulmonary immaturity associated with premature birth and pulmonary surfactant deficiency severe enough to cause respiratory distress syndrome are at increased risk of BPD. Both oxygen and barotrauma play significant roles in the pathogenesis of BPD through oxidant injury and development of epithelial necrosis.

Key Management Requirements

The key areas that require attention in managing an infant with BPD are:

- growth and nutrition
- treatment of ventilation-perfusion mismatch with oxygen and avoiding pulmonary hypertension and cor pulmonale
- aggressive treatment of the reactive airway component
- attention to capillary leak
- the awareness of both the medical and psychosocial stresses placed on a family caring for a child with BPD

In order to accomplish these goals these children must be evaluated on a regular basis, beginning immediately and daily upon discharge.

Nutrition

Children with BPD have metabolic needs far greater than those of the average child. Ultimately, the resolution of BPD requires growth of new lung tissue with development of new alveoli and repair of airways. Compared to the average infant's requirement of 100 calories per kilogram per day, it may take as much as 150 to 175 calories per kilogram daily to meet the metabolic needs of an infant with BPD. Care must be exercised to avoid administering too much fluid in an attempt to provide adequate calories, thereby compromising cardiopulmonary stability.

Providing adequate nutrition to an infant with BPD can be quite frustrating. These children tend to feed poorly due to baseline tachypnea and neurological compromise, and acute pulmonary infections may further complicate feeding. Calorically dense preparations (24-30 calories per ounce of formula) should be used to the limits of the infant's gastrointestinal tract tolerance, with a weight gain goal of 10 to 20 grams per day. Frequently, nasogastric feedings are necessary to meet nutritional needs. If nasogastric feedings are prolonged, placement of a gastrostomy tube should be considered.

Gastroesophageal Reflux

Many infants with BPD have gastroesophageal reflux (GER). GER may compromise not only nutritional status but may lead to aspiration causing further pulmonary compromise. When infants fail to grow or their overall clinical condition deteriorates, the possibility of GER must be investigated. This evaluation should include a thorough history and clinical assessment of the child's eating behavior. It is important to keep in mind that infants may aspirate from above with oral feedings, may aspirate from below if GER is present, or both.

Radiographic studies include an upper gastrointestinal X ray or a technetium-labeled milk scan. If clinically significant GER is suspected, conservative medical management including thickened feedings, placing the child in the prone position, and providing the child with smaller, more frequent feedings should be attempted. Pharmacologic treatment includes antacids and histamine blockers to reduce inflammation of the lower esophageal sphincter in order to improve its function (cimetidine 10 mg/kg/dose q.i.d.); or an agent to tighten the lower esophageal sphincter (metoclopramide 0.1 mg/kg/dose q.i.d.). If these measures are unsuccessful, the child should have a more extensive evaluation, which may include a milk scan or pH probe, and ultimately—if medical management fails—a Nissen fundoplication should be considered.

Prevention of Cor Pulmonale

The fundamental pharmacologic management of BPD is oxygen therapy. The most common error in the management of children with BPD is to discontinue oxygen prematurely. The goal should be to maintain an oxygen saturation of at least 94%. Chronic hypoxemia not only impairs growth and development, but may lead to pulmonary hypertension with the eventual development of right heart failure. Too often infants with BPD present in acute distress with florid cor pulmonale. This is generally preventable and should be avoided at all costs. Oxygen should be continued until the child demonstrates good sleeping oxygen saturations of 92%-94% on a home oximetry study.

Diuretics improve pulmonary mechanics through reducing interstitial edema and increased pulmonary water content and increasing lung compliance, thus reducing the work of breathing. Children on chronic diuretic therapy need careful monitoring for electrolyte imbalances, and routinely require potassium chloride supplements. These children need to be followed closely for the development of renal calculi. Hydrochlorothiazide and spironolactone in combination may be associated with fewer complications than furosemide therapy. Glucocorticoids may be useful in reducing capillary leak and interstitial fluid.

Airways Disease

BPD is characterized by severe damage to the small airways, causing atelectasis and fibrosis. Subsequently, airway reactivity becomes an important factor. Children with BPD often require nebulized bronchodilator therapy consisting of beta agonists (albuterol) and cromolyn (Intal). Chest physiotherapy improves pulmonary toileting, reduces mucus plugging, and decreases the risk of infection. Alternate day glucocorticoids may be necessary to control the reactive component. Intermittent courses of daily glucocorticoids can be used to control acute exacerbations of reactivity often associated with viral infections. Beta agonists may also be beneficial in increasing cilial motility and improving lung clearance.

Central airway lesions are common. There can be a component of subglottic stenosis related to tracheal trauma from chronic intubation. Tracheomalacia or bronchomalacia may occur. This may be related to chronic instrumentation of the airway, chronic inflammation from bacterial colonization, and poor nutrition. However, at this time airway malacia is not well understood. Some children with BPD evidence sudden episodes of severe cyanosis associated with wheezing and marked difficulty in breathing—a "BPD spell" probably related to collapse of central airways during forced expiratory efforts.

Preventing pulmonary infections is very important and contact with individuals with respiratory infections should be avoided. Immunizations should be up to date; the influenza vaccine should be given routinely.

In severe forms of the disease, there can be significant airways obstruction, chronic carbon dioxide retention with pCO_2s of 60 torr, tracheostenosis and severe central airway malacia. These children should be considered for a tracheostomy and chronic mechanical ventilation, which has been demonstrated to improve growth and development. These children can be managed at home on chronic mechanical ventilation.

Other Complications

There are many other associated complications of BPD, and the infant who fails to grow and improve should have a cardiac and GER workup. Children with recurrent infections should be evaluated for hypogammaglobulinemia. Systemic hypertension is a common complication and should be monitored and treated. There is a high incidence of inguinal hernias and middle ear disease as well. Elective surgery should be planned carefully and should not occur during the respiratory virus season. Careful attention must be paid to administration of fluids intra- and postoperatively, as well as to optimizing pulmonary toileting.

Home Equipment Needs

Transition to home can be quite difficult for these families as they often have unrealistic expectations. All patients who require oxygen should be on a cardiac monitor. The tachycardia alarm is helpful as tachycardia is a response to hypoxemia and may indicate the oxygen has become disconnected or oxygen requirements have increased. The parents must be trained in the use of equipment, and they must learn to manage the monitor alarms and the anxiety associated with them. Frequent false alarms are the rule. Families must be trained in cardiopulmonary resuscitation (CPR) with periodic renewal and to recognize early respiratory infections. Respiratory syncytial virus, influenza virus, adenovirus, parainfluenza virus, and other pathogens can cause substantial setbacks in the pulmonary status of these infants. Often hospitalization is required and recovery is generally slow.

In addition to their cardiopulmonary disease, many of these children have visual, auditory, and developmental deficits. Some are behaviorally disorganized, irritable, and generally difficult to manage. As their acute intercurrent illnesses are potentially life threatening, the stress levels in the families can often become enormous; and internal family tension can be created that may be unsolvable as long as the child with BPD remains fragile. Methods for coping with this tension are quite individual, and the health care team must be aware of these issues and must be responsive to cries for help and need for support.

Oxygen, apnea monitoring, home equipment needs, overnight sleep studies, and evaluation of the adequacy of home oxygen therapy via periodic pulse oximetry checks are services that can be provided by durable medical equipment (DME) companies and home health agencies (HHA).

To ensure successful transition into the home setting and its continued success, good relationships with the DME provider and HHA are essential. Most rural areas are covered by a reputable DME company. DME providers and HHA have respiratory therapists who can provide the clinician with another assessment of the child's respiratory status, and they provide ongoing teaching and review of respiratory assessment, treatment, and use of equipment. They can usually provide CPR refresher courses for the family, in many cases in the home setting. When ordering pulse oximetry checks it is necessary to be specific in the data you want collected for the results to be of greatest value. Generally, percentage of oxygen saturation, heart rate, respiratory rate, and general respiratory condition of the child on varying fractions of inspired oxygen including room air provide valuable data to assess oxygen need. Likewise, when ordering overnight oxygen saturation studies, specific parameters must be given as to what is acceptable and when to abort the test if respiratory distress is noted. Generally, these tests and equipment for the child with BPD are covered by third-party reimbursers but may require a detailed letter of medical necessity to ensure coverage and reimbursement.

Consultation Needs

In addition to developing close working relationships with a local DME and HHA, the rural primary care provider must have support from tertiary care specialists and subspecialists. Before the child is discharged from the hospital, it is important to prepare a schedule of follow-up, to outline what should be done at each visit, and to agree on acceptable and unacceptable ranges for follow-up parameters. For example, what weight gain or oxygen saturation levels should prompt a change in therapy or a call to the tertiary care center? A system of tertiary care consultants should be available 24 hours daily to provide advice. To be helpful, the tertiary care advisors must be familiar with the resources and capabilities available in the specific rural setting. Fostering such primary and tertiary care consulting relationships can be difficult, but often this saves families time, money, emotional distress, and may even save lives.

Summary

In summary, BPD is a chronic syndrome consisting of chronic pulmonary insufficiency, airway reactivity, ventilation-perfusion mismatch, poor growth, and a host of associated medical and psychosocial complications. Management should focus on adequate nutrition to ensure growth, oxygenation, bronchodilator therapy, diuretics, and attention to the recognized complications. If these children fail to grow, diagnostic evaluation should be performed. Important psychosocial issues need to be addressed. In rural areas, DME providers and a close relationship with the tertiary care center can be very helpful in monitoring and managing these children.

Recommended Reading

Baley, J. E., Hancharik, S. M., & Rivers, A. (1988). Observations of a support group in parents of children with severe bronchopulmonary dysplasia. *Developmental and Behavioral Pediatrics, 9,* 19-24.
Kao, L. C., Warburton, D., Sargent, C. W., et al. (1983). Furosemide acutely decreases airways resistance in chronic bronchopulmonary dysplasia. *Pediatrics, 103,* 624-629.

60 EXPLORING RURAL MEDICINE

Kurzner, S. I., Garg, M., Bautista, D. B., Bader, D., Meritt, R. J., Warburton, D., & Keens, T. G. (1988). Growth failure in infants with bronchopulmonary dysplasia: Nutrition and elevated resting metabolic expenditure. *Pediatrics, 81,* 379-384.

Motoyama, E. K., Fort, M. D., Klesh, K. W., Mutich, R. L., & Guthrie, R. D. (1987). Early onset of airway reactivity in premature infants with bronchopulmonary dysplasia. *American Review of Respiratory Disease, 136,* 50-57.

Northway, W. H., Rosan, R. C., & Porter, D. Y. (1967). Pulmonary disease following respiratory therapy of hyaline membrane disease: Bronchopulmonary dysplasia. *New England Journal of Medicine, 276,* 357-368.

O'Brodovich, R. M., & Mellins, R. B. (1985). Bronchopulmonary dysplasia. *American Review of Respiratory Disease, 132,* 6942.

Orenstein, S. R. (1990). Prone positioning in infant gastroesophageal reflux: Is elevation of the head worth the trouble? *Journal of Pediatrics, 117,* 184-187.

Werthammer, J., Brown, E. R., Neff, R. K., & Taeusch, H. W. (1982). Sudden infant death syndrome in infancy with BPD. *Pediatrics, 69,* 301-304.

5
■ ■ ■

Attention Deficit-Hyperactivity Disorder

CAROLYN McKAY

Introduction

Behavior, learning problems, and poor school performance are concerns that are often brought to the rural family physician's office for diagnosis, management, and family support. The diagnosis of these disorders is complex and still evolving as an art and a science. Because attention deficit-hyperactivity disorder (ADHD) has been well publicized in professional and lay literature, especially the pharmacological portion of treatment, families may arrive in the office expecting the physician to confirm and fix the problem. Such a quick fix is seldom possible.

The diagnosis of ADHD is not a neatly defined entity with specific criteria that can be checked off a list. It is often a painstaking process of ongoing observation, therapeutic trials, and careful documentation. The primary symptoms of inattention and behavioral impulsivity overlap with aggression and noncompliance. Although frequently accompanied by learning disabilities, ADHD does not necessarily imply academic deficits.

This chapter will outline the methods of diagnosis and the modalities for therapy. ADHD requires the cooperation of a team of health care professionals, educators, and the parents and child. Although at first the process appears overly burdensome and time consuming, management of ADHD is possible in the rural community and can be done with a moderate time commitment from the physician.

Diagnosis

Attention deficit-hyperactivity disorder is established by the documentation of at least 8 of the characteristics listed in Table 5.1. These characteristics should be documented by observations of teachers, physicians, and office staff as well as historical information from the parents.

Medical history, physical examination, and information gathering are used to rule out other possible problems and to create the diagnosis of attention deficit-hyperactivity disorder. Family history from parents, a teacher interview, input from the child, formal child behavior ratings, and behavior ratings by parents and teachers are all needed to complete the diagnostic process.

History

Pertinent history should include the following:

- family history
- preconception maternal history
- pregnancy and delivery history
- childhood illness history
- developmental history
- parenting arrangement history
- parenting style and expectations
- school style and expectations of parents

For the rural family physician, much of this history may already be part of the office records. It is helpful to review the documentation of these events, because memory may be influenced by parental perceptions. If part of the information is not contained in your medical records it is useful to obtain old medical records from outside sources to compare them to the parental perceptions of historical events.

Family history includes the school history of parents and siblings. Use of special education, repeating grades, lack of high school diploma, or history of behavior problems may provide clues. Dyslexia recurs within families at a 35% to 45% rate, compared to the population-based rates of only 3% to 10%. Reading difficulty can

Table 5.1 Criteria for Diagnosing Attention Deficit-Hyperactivity Disorder

A. A disturbance of at least 6 months during which at least eight of the following are present:

   1. Often fidgets with hands or feet or squirms in seat (adolescents may be limited to subjective feelings of restlessness).
   2. Has difficulty remaining seated when required to do so.
   3. Is easily distracted by extraneous stimuli.
   4. Has difficulty awaiting turn in games or group situations.
   5. Often blurts out answers to questions before they have been completed.
   6. Has difficulty following through on instructions from others (not due to oppositional behavior or failure of comprehension).
   7. Has difficulty sustaining attention in tasks or play activities.
   8. Often shifts from one uncompleted activity to another.
   9. Has difficulty playing quietly.
   10. Often talks excessively.
   11. Often interrupts or intrudes on others, for example, intrudes into other children's games.
   12. Often does not seem to listen to what is being said to him or her.
   13. Often loses things necessary for tasks or activities at school or at home (for example, toys, pencils, books, assignments).
   14. Often engages in physically dangerous activities without considering possible consequences (not for the purpose of thrill seeking), for example, runs into street without looking.

B. Onset before the age of 7.

C. Does not meet the criteria for Pervasive Development Disorder, i.e., developmental delays.

SOURCE: From the Diagnostic and Statistical Manual of Mental Disorders, 3rd Ed., Revised (American Psychiatric Association, 1987).

masquerade as inattention, oppositional behavior, or ADHD. The parents' interest in school and support of school performance are often critical elements in the diagnosis of other problems and in management.

Maternal history predating the pregnancy with this child should be elicited. Nutrition status of the mother at conception can be affected by her age and may affect fetal development. Adolescents frequently consume diets high in calories, fat, and salt but low in iron, calcium, and vitamins. Cigarettes, alcohol, and street drug use frequently compromise nutritional status, which affects the vulnerable fetus in the early weeks of gestation. Was mother socially supported during the pregnancy? Depression, loneliness, and isolation tend to affect nutritional status. Information about the pregnancy, labor, and delivery are important but not often diagnostic. Birth weight, gestational age, condition at birth and discharge time may be clues to other problems.

Early development may provide clues about the parents' perceptions of their child—placid, active, attractive, difficult. If the infant was wanted and met parents' expectations in eating, sleeping, and growing, a line of inquiry ends. History of illness in early childhood and developmental milestones should be checked.

It is always useful to inquire about why medical advice was sought at this time. Parents, relatives, neighbors, or a teacher may believe the child has a problem. Explore the concerns to identify who owns the problem and its implications. This often starts a therapeutic plan that must meet the most concerned individual's need if it is to be successful.

History from a teacher might be obtained by telephone and should include samples of daily work, general behavioral observations, and information regarding the type of classroom setting and number of other students in that room.

History provided by the child allows you to measure his or her perception of reality against adult reports and to begin to understand the impact of the reported problem on the child's motivation, self-esteem in school and at home.

Physical Examination

Physical evaluation must include:

- plotted height, weight, and head circumference since birth
- vision and hearing screening
- general body habitus, especially facies
- speech—articulation, vocabulary, fluency, and understanding
- neurological evaluation—coordination, handedness, gross motor, fine motor, quality of movements

The physical assessment of a child suspected of having ADHD is similar to any thorough examination, with emphasis on eyes, ears, speech, and neurological function. The growth pattern may show intra- and extrauterine growth retardation. Thyroid dysfunction may be uncovered by observation of growth. Surprisingly, parents and teachers may complain of behavioral problems when a child is treated for hypothyroidism and becomes more active.

While perusing the child's growth pattern, consider that a child who is very small may have been infantilized by caregivers and parents. When such a child encounters the school system, the picking up, carrying, and doing for the child that has occurred throughout life may have created behavior patterns that interfere with independent learning. At the other end of the growth curve, a child who is taller and heavier than age mates will face expectations beyond those appropriate for age. A 35-pound 2-year-old will have limited speech, probably will not be toilet trained, and will exhibit 2-year-old testing behavior but may look like a 4-year-old physically. Keep chronologic age in mind and verify that the environment is supportive and patient.

Can the child see and hear normally? Hearing loss and moderate visual impairment characteristically are diagnosed late by medical professionals. Parents may deny the problem. Testing can require specialist consultation. Children of any age can be evaluated by a skilled ophthalmologist or optometrist for vision, although several visits may be required. Hearing can be evaluated depending on age by brainstem evoked response, skilled conditioned behavioral observation, or audiometer, again possibly requiring more than one visit. Abnormal tympanometry can provide a clue that hearing may be impaired but this test itself does not measure hearing. A family history of hearing loss, prematurity, treatment with ototoxic antibiotics, prolonged intubation, recurrent or persistent ear infections, or abnormal facial structure may be clues to hearing problems. Children with midface hypoplasia such as Down syndrome or fetal alcohol syndrome (FAS) have increased risk of ear and sinus infections and therefore hearing problems.

Listen to the child's speech and observe the play pattern. A very bright child may chatter or converse with sentence structure and vocabulary beyond age expectation. This may upset a conventional classroom. A child with a history of central nervous system problems such as shunted hydrocephalus may chatter in a stylized social pattern without much content. This occasionally is misinterpreted as strong verbal skills and creates academic expectations beyond the intellectual capacity of the child.

When observing the child's head and neck consider ear position and configuration, mid face development, placement of eyes, length of philtrum, and development of the jaw. Down syndrome and FAS show mid face hypoplasia and are associated with many school and behavioral problems. Look for other signs of dysmorphology, such as unusual proportions of any body parts. Are the arm span and height well matched? Look at the hands. Are the nails normal, dermatographics as expected, fingers symmetric? Are chest and abdomen normal? Degenerative metabolic disease may provide physical clues to their diagnoses. Examine the genitalia for the enlarged testicles found in fragile X syndrome.

Neurological examination can be done with the child playing or attempting a task in your exam room or the waiting room. Consider the quality of gross and fine motor activity. Is muscle tone increased or decreased? Is there asymmetry in use of the limbs? Is strength normal? Is there an abnormally strong preference for one hand? Is grasp pattern normal for age? Prenatal stroke may show subtle manifestations when seen at preschool or school age but can impair expected performance. Cerebral palsy may manifest itself by a tendency to toe-walk or excessive fisting or abnormal grasp of a pencil. Sydenham's chorea with involuntary movements can present as inability to sit still and may be perceived as hyperactivity. Is sitting posture normal? Can the child get from sitting to standing normally? Can he hop, skip, ride a bike at the expected age? Many very active boys can balance and ride a two-wheeled bike at 5 or 6 years, but have neither the interest nor the fine motor skills to master writing.

Performance and Academic Evaluation

Evaluate the child's fund of knowledge. Is it age appropriate? It is useful to check periodically on what is age appropriate. If knowledge is not age appropriate consider why not. Does the home provide appropriate verbal patterning? Is the child living in a multilingual household? Is the television on continually? Who converses with the child? What does the parent believe is appropriate verbal interaction? Be aware that a single parent or two working parents may have very few hours of interaction with a rested, receptive child. Some child-care settings may warehouse children, providing little appropriate language or behavior patterning.

Gather information about parent and teacher expectations. A very active child in a quiet family may appear unusual. A child of normal intelligence in an intellectually gifted family may be judged slow. A child with intellectually limited parents may have had limited learning opportunities. A child who determines his own rhythm at home with accommodating parents may be a misfit in a very structured classroom.

A child who performs well in some areas may be perceived to be a behavior problem for not performing in other areas. Check the level of reading skills. Some children read well mechanically but cannot comprehend material. By third or fourth grade this impedes class work. Computation may exceed math comprehension or vice versa. Difficulty in forming letters or words may impair classroom writing performance. An eager, bright child who wishes to please may memorize or use contextual clues to mask deficits, for example, memorize the visual acuity chart from students ahead in line and therefore "pass" the eye test.

Academic information is essential for the formulation of the diagnosis of ADHD. It is important to have a systematic way of obtaining, recording, and summarizing this information. The ANSER system (Excelsior Publishing Company, Cambridge, Massachusetts) is one method of organizing the needed academic information. It is a standard format that may be familiar to your education colleagues and will simplify the data gathering for you. The ANSER system includes data on all academic areas such as reading comprehension, reading rate, word analysis skills, spelling, arithmetic facts, arithmetic concepts, letter formation in writing, musical skills, and artistic ability. In addition, performance areas such as playing sports, mechanical skills, and coordination are included. Other major areas to be assessed are language, visual-perceptual function, memory, and temporal-sequential organization; and the questionnaire also assesses motivation, imagination, creativity, sense of humor, and enthusiasm.

Each of these categories is evaluated and recorded for typical performance as strong for age, appropriate for age, delayed 1 year or delayed more than 1 year. In addition, the variability of the child's day-to-day performance is assessed and recorded as consistent performance, somewhat variable, or highly variable. Completion of the ANSER grid provides a very complete assessment of a child's school ability and is an important portion of the diagnostic and follow-up process.

It is necessary for most of us to seek help from skilled colleagues in the evaluation of children with learning or behavior problems. It is not unusual for ADHD to be accompanied by other problems. Treatment will not be successful until all aspects of the problem have been identified and treatment has been devised for the total package of issues. Several different types of professionals may be helpful. The school psychologist may be able to provide objective data on academic performance and presumed intellectual capacity. Marked differences from one subtest to another subtest and performance scores less than verbal scores in a given area may point to learning problems. Be aware that the specific test chosen by a school may determine that a child is within the range of normal when other standardized tests will better demonstrate deficits or problems. The ideal consultant should be objective from the child's vantage point, and should have available a wide repertoire of tests including those that could be used for a physically handicapped, hearing handicapped, or non-English-speaking child.

Other helpful professionals are neurologists; developmental pediatricians; geneticists; family counselors who are accustomed to using behavior modification; audiologists; educational specialists who know the local school system, available teaching modalities, and curricula; and legal mandates experts. Although these professionals may not be easily available in the local community, most states require the school system to provide education testing from visiting consultants or by referral to regional centers. Most university hospitals or clinics provide a multidisciplinary clinic for those children who are very difficult to diagnose and treat.

Treatment

Even if no specific contributing factors can be found for the behavior of concern, changing that behavior is the usual goal. The child's self-image, the parents' self-confidence, and the teacher's professional ability are all important factors to consider when modifying a behavior that disturbs a child's school life.

The physician's role encompasses the historical and physical examination, data collection, and also case management. Demystifying the diagnosis for child, parent, and teacher can allow fruitful planning for change. Strategies to bypass or minimize deficits can be made. Specific therapy for the child or parent may be needed. Medication may be indicated and will require monitoring. Coordination of diagnosis, interpretation to various other professionals, and advocacy for the child remain physician and health care team responsibilities.

Behavior change may be brought about by a variety of therapies. Setting priorities allows realistic goals. Improved communication between parent and teacher may allow the parents to reinforce school expectation. Review or practice of academic skills or material at home may assist in classroom success. Increased rest or appropriate meals may help the child perform. Consistent discipline methods may redirect energy both at home and school.

Readjustment of academic goals, tutoring, and the use of multiple learning modalities may be useful. Reduction of distracting environmental input can help some children focus attention. Use of a study carrel, resituating the child's desk in a different part of the classroom, and small class size may be useful.

Drug Therapy

Stimulant medications for attention deficit disorder can improve concentration and diminish impulsivity. The most commonly prescribed drugs are methylphenidate (Ritalin), dextroamphetamine (Dexedrine), and pemoline (Cylert). These medications can be prescribed only by physicians, not teachers or psychologists. Because the drugs have potential value as street drugs careful documentation of the indications, amounts, and monitoring of the children is important.

Drug therapy is sometimes initiated with very high expectations of success by parents and teachers. Although drug therapy has well-documented positive effects for some children, it is not uniformly effective. Documentation of classroom behavior before initiating a drug is essential, and periodic monitoring must be performed to support ongoing use of medication. Use of on-task behavior checklists (Figure 5.1) by the teacher can guide decision making in adjusting dosages as well.

Dextroamphetamine is a Schedule II drug. Dosage for children 3 to 5 years of age starts at 2 to 5 milligrams daily. For children 6 and older, dosage is begun at 5 milligrams daily. The dosage can be

Student_____ Teacher_____ Date_____

#	Question	0-49%	50-69%	70-79%	80-89%	90-100%
1.	Estimate the percentage of written math work completed (regardless of accuracy) relative to classmates.	0-49%	50-69%	70-79%	80-89%	90-100%
2.	Estimate the percentage of written language arts work completed (regardless of accuracy) relative to classmates	0-49%	50-69%	70-79%	80-89%	90-100%
3.	Estimate the accuracy of the completed written math work (percentage of correct work done)	0-49%	50-69%	70-79%	80-89%	90-100%
4.	Estimate the accuracy of written language arts work (percentage of correct work done)	0-49%	50-69%	70-79%	80-89%	90-100%
5.	How consistent has this child's academic performance been over the past week?	highly variable 1	variable 2	somewhat consistent 3	consistent 4	very consistent 5
6.	How frequently does the student accurately follow teacher instructions or class discussion during large group instruction?	never 1	rarely 2	sometimes 3	often 4	very often 5
7.	How frequently does the student accurately follow teacher instructions or class discussion during small group instruction?	never 1	rarely 2	sometimes 3	often 4	very often 5
8.	How quickly does this child learn new material?	very slow 1	slow 2	average 3	quickly 4	very quickly 5
9.	What is the quality or neatness of the child's handwriting?	poor 1	fair 2	average 3	above average 4	excellent 5
10.	How often does the child complete written work in a careless, hasty fashion?	never 1	rarely 2	sometimes 3	often 4	very often 5
11.	How frequently does the child take more time to complete work than his/her classmates?	never 1	rarely 2	sometimes 3	often 4	very often 5
12.	How often is the child able to pay attention without your prompting him/her?	never 1	rarely 2	sometimes 3	often 4	very often 5
13.	How frequently does the child require your assistance to accurately complete his/her academic work?	never 1	rarely 2	sometimes 3	often 4	very often 5
14.	How often does the child begin written work prior to understanding the directions?	never 1	rarely 2	sometimes 3	often 4	very often 5
15.	How often does the child appear to be staring excessively or "spaced" out?	never 1	rarely 2	sometimes 3	often 4	very often 5
16.	How often does the child withdraw or tend to lack an emotional response in a social situation?	never 1	rarely 2	sometimes 3	often 4	very often 5

Figure 5.1. Children's Learning Profile

70

increased incrementally to a total of 40 milligrams daily, which may be given in one or two doses. This drug has the potential for causing insomnia, anorexia, and many other side effects. Extreme psychological dependence can occur.

Methylphenidate should not be used in children under six years of age. The usual dosage is 5 milligrams before breakfast and lunch, swallowed as a whole tablet because it is time released. Dosage is adjusted to a total of no more than 60 milligrams per day, although 20 milligrams is the usual total dose. If a 1 month trial does not demonstrate effectiveness, the drug should be discontinued. Side effects of insomnia and possible growth suppression can occur as well as other varied complaints.

Pemoline is chemically unrelated to amphetamine and methylphenidate. It has not been shown to have a potential for abuse. The usual dosage begins with 37.5 milligrams daily and is raised by 18.75 milligrams each week until effectiveness is noted. In contrast to methylphenidate and amphetamines, behavioral change is gradual and may require 3 to 4 weeks to be noticeable. Pemoline can cause insomnia, growth suppression, and liver dysfunction. Liver enzymes should be checked monthly at first and then quarterly.

Summary

The most important function of the physician is to advocate for the child in creating the most appropriate home and school setting. In addition, it is important to support the parents in providing discipline, supervision, and learning opportunities for their child. The school may need help to facilitate learning.

Recommended Reading

Abikoff, H., Gittelman-Klein, R., & Klein, D. (1977). Validation of a classroom observation code for hyperactive children. *Journal of Consulting and Clinical Psychology, 45,* 772-783.

American Psychiatric Association. (1987). *Diagnostic and statistical manual of mental disorders* (3rd ed., rev.). Washington, DC: Author.

Guevremont, D. C., DuPaul, G. J., & Bakley, R. A. (1990). Diagnosis and assessment of attention deficit-hyperactivity disorder in children. *Journal of School Psychology, 28,* 51-79.

Halperin, J. M., Wolf, L. E., & Pascualvaca, D. M. (1988). Differential assessment of attention and impulsivity in children. *Journal of the American Academy of Child and Adolescent Psychiatry, 23,* 285-290.

Kendall, P. C., & Braswell, L. (1985). *Cognitive-behavior therapy for impulsive children.* New York: Guilford Press.

Klorman, R., Trumaghim, J. T., & Salzman, L. F. (1988). Effects of methylphenidate on attention-deficit hyperactivity disorder with and without aggressive/non-compliant features. *Journal of Abnormal Psychology, 97,* 413-422.

Levine, M. D. (1992). Attentional variation and dysfunction. In M. D. Levine, W. B. Carey, & A. C. Crocker (Eds.), *Developmental-behavioral pediatrics* (2nd ed.). Philadelphia: W. B. Saunders.

Levine, M. D. (1992). Learning disorders: their elucidation and management. *Pediatric Basics, 62,* 10-15.

Other Resources

Children With Attention Deficit Disorders
499 NW 70th Avenue, Suite 308
Plantation, FL 33324
305-587-3700

Foundation for Children With Learning Disabilities
99 Park Avenue
New York, NY 10016
212-686-7211

Learning Disabilities Association of America
4158 Library Road
Pittsburgh, PA 15234
412-341-1515

Orton Dyslexia Society
724 York Road
Baltimore, MD 21204
301-296-0232

6
■ ■ ■

Recognition and Evaluation of Child Abuse

DANIEL D. BROUGHTON

Introduction

Child abuse is a long-standing problem that dates back to the earliest recorded history. Although there is clear evidence of child maltreatment in this country from the time of the first settlers, there was no coordinated effort in this area by the medical community until the early 1960s, when C. Henry Kempe coined the term *battered child syndrome*. Since then great strides have been made both in recognizing and in dealing with this problem. As a part of this increased awareness and deeper understanding, physicians and other health care providers are now required to file a report of suspected child abuse to the appropriate state agency, so that appropriate intervention can be promptly instituted and further suffering by the child can be avoided.

The actual incidence of child abuse is not clear because of the secrecy surrounding the problem and the difficulty in identifying many of the cases. It is estimated that there are 685,000 cases of physical child abuse and neglect each year. Experts dealing with child sexual abuse indicate that at least 1 in 4 girls and 1 in 8 boys will have an abusive or exploitive episode before their 18th birthday.

Developing an exact definition of child abuse is difficult because of the complexity of the issue. Every state has passed legislation to deal with the problem but each defines it somewhat differently. All include the same basic elements:

- nonaccidental injury
- neglect
- sexual molestation
- mental injury

Other components of the problem also play significant roles. An act of omission, such as the failure to protect a child by leaving him or her in a potentially abusive or dangerous situation, can be as serious a risk to a child as an episode where the perpetrator actually strikes at the child. Likewise, a threat to a child may be as damaging as the act itself by leaving a child frightened and insecure.

Some concern may be raised that normal but strict discipline might inappropriately be considered as child abuse, but there are clear distinctions between them. Abuse usually is the result of anger or loss of control by the abuser, without the clear goal of discipline. Generally, abusive acts will lead the child to alter behavior out of fear, often leaving a damaged self-esteem. The child may not have a normal, nurturing relationship with the abuser, which may lead to difficulty in learning how to interact with others. On the other hand, discipline is clearly aimed at misbehavior and intends to give the child a realization that a particular behavior was incorrect or in need of improvement, but will leave self-esteem intact and will help the child develop good social skills.

Evaluation of Possible Child Abuse

The approach to a child who may have been abused is the same as one would apply to any other medical problem. One should take a thorough history, perform a complete physical examination, and use the laboratory as needed to gain further information. After the initial evaluation for suspicion of abuse is entertained, consultation with an expert in the field should be sought, which may include an official child abuse report.

History

As in other medical conditions, the history may well provide the most important clues to an ultimate diagnosis of suspected child abuse. Care needs to be taken to describe any injury, to include how it happened, when it occurred, and where it happened. Differences in the history between reporters (e.g., the child and the parent) should be noted. Conversely, concern may be aroused if the stories sound contrived or rehearsed.

It is essential that behavioral and social matters be probed. Although no specific behavior is pathognomonic for abuse, some behaviors certainly are more concerning than others. For example, an abused child may be either unusually timid or inappropriately friendly. In this way the child may be trying to avoid abuse by staying out of sight or avoiding contact with a potential abuser, or by trying to "get on the good side of the abuser." Complaints by a child about having been beaten or hit should be pursued vigorously, as should comments indicating that the child is afraid of his or her care givers.

Sexual abuse is often difficult to identify because it is not considered and there is a reluctance by most physicians to deal with it if it is brought up. Comments about inappropriate or unwanted sexual advances by adults must be taken very seriously. Likewise, outward sexual or seductive behavior by a child should alert the medical provider to the possibility of sexual abuse. Although difficult for most medical providers, it is important that any discussion of possible sexual abuse must be warm and supportive. Care must be taken not to show anger or revulsion that may be interpreted by the child as directed at him or her. Failure to deal with the issue at this time may give the child a clear message not to talk about it, thus reinforcing secrecy. When sexual abuse is considered, the child should be asked if he or she was photographed or videotaped. The use of such equipment by abusers has become common.

Abuse often occurs in families with high stress levels. Therefore, family situations such as financial difficulties, marital discord, drug or alcohol misuse should be probed as part of the social history. Other stressful situations, such as twins or triplets and chronic illness in a family, which clearly are not the "fault" of the family, also are associated with an increased incidence of child abuse. Because many abusive parents were abused as children, questions regarding the parents' upbringing may provide valuable insight.

The child's past medical history often provides important clues as well. Some health problems may mimic abuse, such as bleeding disorders. A history of significant injuries may reveal a pattern suggestive of abuse. Even the absence of a history of trauma may be important when evidence of significant trauma is subsequently found during the physical exam or on X-ray evaluation.

A final important step is to confirm the past medical history by obtaining copies of previous medical records. Refusal by a parent or guardian to such a request should immediately alert a care provider that a problem may exist. On one hand it may be an attempt to conceal evidence of prior abuse; but also, a request for old records may help to identify children who are missing. Whether taken illegally by a non-family member or a parent, the child may be unable or afraid to provide his or her real identity. A record check or a refusal to permit it may be the only clue.

Physical Examination

As is true in all medical problems, the physical examination should begin with an accurate recording of the vital signs to include height and weight measurements. They may provide a valuable clue to chronic or severe abuse by showing inadequate growth or weight loss. The general assessment should include overall appearance and demeanor of the child including apparent mood and level of consciousness. Any unusual behavior or inappropriate responses are also important.

A detailed description of each injury should be made and must include measurements of the bruise, laceration, or other lesion. The location of each lesion must be documented. Bruises or scrapes in areas that children frequently strike during routine falls and activities, such as around the eye or the lower legs, are generally not suggestive of abuse. Other bruises such as on the cheeks, the trunk, or the buttocks are more suggestive of having been struck. The appearance and color of bruises may help indicate when the injury actually occurred. Bruises at different sites may appear to be at different stages of resolution, thus indicating that they occurred at different times. Certain shaped bruises may be highly suspicious. The classic hand print is made up of linear red marks parallel to each other resulting from stretching of skin between the fingers during a slap. Bruises in the shape of an object like a belt or cord also generally indicate abuse. In looking for cutaneous manifestations of abuse it is imperative to examine covered areas of the body, such as under a shirt or shorts, looking for further evidence of injury.

Injuries to the musculoskeletal system also are frequently seen in abused children. Findings may include tenderness, limitation of motion of a joint, hesitation to use an extremity, swelling, or redness.

In addition to the more obvious findings mentioned above, less common but potentially serious injuries must be considered as well. Intracranial injury can be quite subtle on presentation, but devastating to the child if missed. Evaluation of the central nervous system must include a thorough, careful funduscopic examination (looking for evidence of trauma such as retinal hemorrhage) as well as a thorough neurologic examination. The chest wall and the capacity for abdominal organs to move with trauma provide some protection from injury with blunt trauma. However, serious internal injuries such as ruptured spleen or liver, renal hematoma, and hemorrhage into the omentum can occur as a result of child abuse, and need to be considered while completing the physical exam.

In cases where sexual abuse is a possibility, the genitalia should be examined by looking for evidence of acute trauma such as lacerations, abrasions, or bruising. However, it is best not to further traumatize a sexual abuse victim by performing a complete gynecologic or rectal exam under less than ideal conditions. It is best to defer a more detailed exam to someone with considerable experience in evaluating sexual abuse victims, unless time is a critical factor as in the case of an acute assault. When the exam must be done immediately and an expert trained in sexual assault evaluation is not available, care must be taken to perform it with sensitivity. It is essential to follow all of the legal requirements needed for the collection of evidence, and for materials to be carefully collected to avoid contamination. Most hospitals and emergency rooms have a protocol and specimen kits to accomplish this.

Even with careful, thorough examination, in most instances of sexual abuse there will be no evidence of outward injury or trauma. It is common, even with long-term ongoing sexual abuse, for the genital exam to be completely normal. Thus it is impossible for a physician ever completely to rule out sexual abuse.

In addition to careful documentation in the medical record, a final documentation of the visual findings should be made utilizing high quality photographs. Sketches showing the extent of the injury may be helpful but lack the clarity and impact of photographs.

Laboratory Evidence

The use of the laboratory in the evaluation of child abuse has a limited but important role. Tests should be ordered only when they are medically indicated or when there is a specific question to be answered.

Probably the most commonly useful radiologic test is a skeletal screen looking for evidence of fractures. This is particularly true when multiple fractures in different stages of healing are identified. Ultrasound, computerized tomography, magnetic resonance imaging, and radionuclide studies also may be helpful in specific instances, such as looking for intracranial injury, other internal injuries, or early bone changes indicative of recent or subtle injury.

Bleeding studies including platelet count may be needed to evaluate bleeding status in cases of bruising. Other blood and urine studies may be useful when looking for internal injury such as to the liver, spleen, or kidney. Drug screens may be indicated if the misuse of medication or illegal drugs is a possibility. In cases of sexual abuse cultures of the throat, genitalia, and rectum should be considered in symptomatic children.

What to Do When Suspicious

Once there is suspicion that child abuse may have occurred, a report must be made to the appropriate authority. This report is required both legally and for the protection of the child. Although there is some variation among the states, physicians and other professionals involved in caring for patients, such as nurses, technicians, and emergency medical personnel, are designated as mandatory reporters and must file a report in all cases where a *suspicion* of abuse exists. The same laws provide protection to those required to report from subsequent civil legal action as long as the report is made in good faith.

The report, which is to be made to law enforcement and/or to social services, should be made immediately by phone with a written report to follow as soon as possible, usually within 24 hours. In cases of suspected neglect there may be more flexibility with the timing of a report, but it should be filed as quickly as possible. It is not necessary to discuss the report with the family before filing it. However, although confrontation with an accusation is not a good idea, it often is helpful to discuss the findings with the family, explaining the legal and ethical need to report, and to try to work with the family during the ordeal. Often families will understand the need for this action, and sometimes they will even be appreciative.

Reporting to one's supervisor or to the patient's physician may be advisable for information purposes, but does not constitute a valid child abuse report. Once suspicion has been established, the reporting obligation does not change because someone else disagrees with the report, or feels that more proof is needed.

Many physicians have been hesitant to file child abuse reports because of concern over the loss of office time due to court appearances. Most cases of child abuse are settled without involving the physician in court testimony. In those few cases where an appearance is necessary, the court usually will be as cooperative as possible in accommodating the physician's schedule, and the court will reimburse the physician for the time spent testifying.

Once the report has been filed, it becomes the responsibility of law enforcement or social services to determine the risk to the child and to develop a short-term plan. Often this determination is made with the assistance of the physician making the report or with the child's primary care provider. In low-risk situations the child may be released to the parents with appropriate follow-up specifically arranged. If the child is felt to be at risk, the alleged perpetrator should be removed from the home as a first choice. If this is not possible, the child should be placed out of the home with a relative, close friend, or appropriately trained foster parents. As a last resort, hospitalization may be considered, although except in extraordinary situations this step should be limited to those instances where medically indicated.

A long-term plan will then be developed, usually by a multidisciplinary team sanctioned by the county or state, and made up of representatives from medicine, social services, public health, law enforcement, and the courts. This plan may include criminal prosecution, family court proceedings, and/or a long-term family-oriented treatment program. Frequently the child's primary care provider will be involved in this process at some level. The child's physician will know the family, and can be extremely helpful in determining the specific interventions to be recommended, which may include individual or family therapy, parenting education, and a variety of family assistance programs. Subsequent close follow-up and continued medical care is essential. Continuing this care with the primary health provider helps to provide both continuity and stability. Ongoing involvement of the appropriate state agency also is necessary in order to assure that the long-term plan is followed completely.

Special Rural Concerns

In rural practice most children and families are known to most of the providers. It is often difficult to include child abuse as part of the differential diagnosis of an injured child whose care you have provided since birth. Alternatively, certain families may trigger concerns out of proportion to the presenting problem. Such families are often those with lifestyles that appear unhealthy or unusual to the provider.

Knowing the health and religious practices of all groups in your community is important. A southeast Asian child who has bruises over every rib may have been treated at home with "coining" in an attempt to cure the illness for which the provider is seeing the patient. Coining is performed by rubbing the edge of a coin along the ribs repeatedly to relieve chest congestion. The resultant marks may resemble flogging marks to the unwary provider. Indian, African American, or Cajun rituals can appear to be abusive if not understood in the context of the child's ethnic and cultural background.

When abuse does occur, reporting to law enforcement and social services may prove frustrating and futile. Many county sheriffs are elected officials with little or no training in child abuse cases. They are often reluctant to deal with domestic issues such as child physical or sexual abuse.

Rural social service agencies and public health services are overburdened and understaffed. They seldom employ minority workers who may have skills in understanding and dealing with people of similar ethnic backgrounds. Rural counties often pay lower wages than urban centers and are more likely to get young inexperienced personnel.

One solution is to develop a local or county-wide child protection team. The team should have representatives of all disciplines that work with children, including law enforcement, social services, mental health agencies, teachers, physicians, public health nurses, and perhaps clergy. The team should meet regularly not only to educate themselves about child maltreatment problems, but also to learn to understand and to trust the functions of the other agencies. A child protection team can provide guidance and support for the responsible officials and health providers in the initial evaluation, investigation, and emergency disposition of the child.

The evaluation of any child with major trauma or suspected sexual abuse can be supplemented by consultation with a child abuse expert. These cases are most likely to proceed through the legal system, and intervention may hinge on the testimony of an expert witness. The Children's Defense Fund can provide the name of an expert in your region.

Like many other problems, child abuse presents as a spectrum encompassing minor physical or psychological injury to life threatening trauma. And as with any other clinical issue, the rural physician must be prepared to make an initial assessment and then either provide further evaluation and treatment or referral to an appropriate consultant. A missed diagnosis of child maltreatment can have consequences as serious as missing a breast lump or a myocardial infarction.

Summary

The most important goal in child abuse intervention is to keep the child safe and to prevent further abuse. However, in the majority of instances the long-term goal should be to keep the family intact and safe for the child. Long-term foster care or termination of parental rights should be limited to extreme cases.

Recommended Reading

Hager, A., & Emmons, H. (1992). *Evaluation of the sexually abused child: A medical text book and photographic atlas.* New York: Oxford University Press.

Ludwig, S. (1992). *Child abuse medical reference* (2nd ed.). New York: Churchill-Livingston.

MacFarlane, K., & Waterman, J. (1986). *Sexual abuse of young children*. New York: Guilford Press.

Newberger, E. H. (1982). *Child abuse*. Boston: Little, Brown.

Reece, R. M. (1993). *Child abuse: Medical diagnosis and management*. Philadelphia: Lea & Febiger.

7

■ ■ ■

Adolescent Pregnancies in Rural America:

A Review of the Literature and Strategies for Prevention

BARBARA P. YAWN

ROY A. YAWN

Introduction

Each year in the United States more than one million girls under the age of 19 conceive children. Of these pregnant girls, about 40% will choose elective abortions; at least 13% will experience spontaneous abortions (miscarriages); and 95% of the rest will keep their child within its family of origin (Hayes, 1987; McAnarney & Hendee, 1989a). Adolescent pregnancy is a problem that is not unique to the urban or inner-city population. At least 20% of teen births are in rural adolescents (Hayes, 1987). It is certainly not a new problem, and some studies suggest that it is not even a growing problem (Raines, 1991). Why has this issue become a national priority and in some areas a crusade? There are several explanations for the recent upsurge in national interest. Pregnant teens are a high-risk group. They experience high rates of preterm deliveries; they have difficulty fulfilling the important role of parenting; and they are at high risk of poverty in adulthood. Prevention of teen pregnancy requires intervention in early adolescence, preferably before the initiation of sexual activity.

Rural physicians are an important part of the team that educates, cares for, and influences adolescents and their sexual and health decisions. Seldom can sufficient change be implemented through the usual medical care sought by teens from physicians' offices. Adolescent pregnancy is a medical and social issue and requires broad-based community awareness, planning, and intervention. A rural physician need not be the leader in planning community intervention, but without strong support from well-informed, nonjudgmental health providers it is unlikely that any successful program will be developed and maintained. Rural physicians must choose their roles carefully and educate themselves to assure that they can fill them.

The Scope of Teen Sexual Activity

Information has been collected and reported for many years on the sexual activity of urban teens, particularly in the inner cities. Since 1976 information has been available on some selected groups of nonurban teens (Hofferth, 1987c). Comparisons of rates of sexual activity between rural and urban teens have varied. Some studies have found that metropolitan teens were more likely than rural teens to report having had intercourse at least once (Raines, 1991). Others found no significant difference; and one report described an increase in sexual experience in young women from "smaller" communities (Aneshensel, Becerra, Fielder, & Schuler, 1990). The socioeconomic status and racial diversity of urban and rural teens can differ dramatically and must be considered when interpreting these comparison studies.

Detailed information is available from one survey of teens still in high school in a rural Minnesota community (Yawn & Yawn, 1987) and from a study done at the same time from a cross-section of all Minnesota teens (Blum, 1988). The rural study showed that by the twelfth grade, 36.9% of boys and 52.4% of girls had had sexual intercourse; this represented 38.1% of all the students in the high school. At the same time Blum reported that 64% of twelfth grade boys and girls in his broad Minnesota sample said that they had had intercourse. By comparison, Zelnik and Kantner (1980) reported that, in metropolitan teens aged 15 to 19, 42.3% had sexual intercourse before marriage, with an average age of first intercourse of

16.4 years. In the rural study cited here, about one half of sexually active girls had first intercourse at ages 15 to 16.

In Yawn's rural Minnesota group, about 27% of the sexually active teens said that they had regular intercourse; and 27.2% of boys and 11.7% of girls claimed that they had five or more sexual partners. Of the urban girls studied by Zelnik and Kantner (1980), 7% related that they had four to five sexual partners and 8.9% said that they had six or more partners. Intercourse began at the junior high school level for many teens in the rural survey, with about 21% of boys and girls beginning intercourse at ages 13 to 14. Notably, 11.3% of boys and 2.3% of girls said that they were 12 years old or less when they first had intercourse.

Blum cited a rate of contraceptive use by teens of 80%, but about one fifth of the respondents used the withdrawal method. Contraceptives were used at least part of the time by 76.1% of boys and 79.9% of girls in Yawn's study. Zelnik and Kantner (1980) found that 76% of the urban youth in their study used contraceptives at least part of the time.

Yawn's rural Minnesota study was done in a community that is primarily Caucasian, with less than 15% of its residents at or below 200% of the poverty level, and with a large and vocal fundamental religious population. It confirmed that teen sexual activity in rural areas is prevalent at a rate not significantly different from the national averages for white teens. Rural America has not escaped the problems of early teen sexual intercourse, which can lead to unwanted and unplanned pregnancies.

Prevention of teen pregnancies is possible at several levels (McAnarney & Hendee, 1989b). Primary prevention seeks to delay involvement in sexual activity. Secondary prevention focuses on the use of contraceptives in sexually active teens. Tertiary prevention is aimed at preventing teen parenthood, including adoption and abortion. Only primary and secondary prevention will be discussed here.

Conceptualization

The problems of adolescent sexual intercourse and pregnancy are very complex. Many factors may reinforce or interdict these activities. Factors to be considered here include biology and maturation;

social influences; race, cultural, and economic factors; media exposure; the role of parents; peer environments and dating behavior;
personality and self-esteem; perception of risk and benefit; and
societal trends.

Biology and Maturation

Both boys and girls attain biologic maturity at an earlier age than
did preceding generations (Donovan, 1990). Estrogen and progesterone levels in adolescent girls are positively related to interest
in sexual activity. Postpubertal testosterone levels of boys corre-
late positively with interest and participation in sexual intercourse
(Udry, Billy, Morris, Gorff, & Raj, 1985; Udry, Talbert, & Morris,
1986). However, about 61% of sexually active black boys experience
first intercourse prior to puberty (Hofferth, 1987c).

The role of the appearance of secondary sexual characteristics has
not been defined. Do young teens who appear more "adult-like"
experience earlier first intercourse? Gender roles appear to be defined differently because females are more likely to be "in a long-
term relationship" when they first have intercourse, whereas 50% of
boys report their first intercourse to be with a "friend" or casual
acquaintance (Zelnick & Shah, 1983).

Social Influences

Where a teen lives is very important in determining the age and
circumstances of initiation of intercourse. However, merely defining the area as urban or rural is not sufficiently descriptive. Characteristics of the community that do influence the rate of sexual activity in unmarried teenagers include poverty, structure and mix of the
community by socioeconomic status, ethnic factors, and strength of
religious beliefs (Billy, Rodgers, & Udry, 1984). Ethnic isolation is
more likely to be found in rural communities. Isolated black communities have a higher fraction of teenagers who have engaged in
sexual intercourse than well-integrated, racially mixed communities (Humenick, Wilkerson, & Paul, 1991). This may suggest that
community intervention is more appropriate in the socially isolated
rural areas.

The presence of strong religious beliefs (not merely church attendance) has been shown to delay the age of initiation of sexual

activity (Jessor, Costa, Jessor, & Donovan, 1983; Zelnik, Kantner, & Ford, 1981). Physicians in rural areas can be instrumental in helping churches recognize their own community's problems with adolescent sexuality and pregnancy. Community task forces to prevent teen sexual activity and pregnancy should include representation from church groups.

Race, Cultural, and Economic Factors

Black adolescents initiate intercourse at a younger age than whites irrespective of socioeconomic status. Hispanic adolescents also are more likely to be sexually active than are white teens, but they are also more likely to be married (Hofferth, 1987c). Cultural factors (Swenson, Erickson, Ehlinger, Carlson, & Swaney, 1989) and perceived career opportunities may influence the racial variations in onset of sexual activity. The career options listed by black women were fewer than those of white women at all socioeconomic levels and may influence desire for earlier motherhood (Ensminger, 1987). Rural communities often have fewer visible career options for all adolescents. Increasing the awareness of career and educational choices may be helpful in delaying participation in sexual intercourse (Watson & Kelly, 1990).

Media Exposure

No studies have shown that exposure to sexually explicit materials on television is a causative factor for earlier or increased sexual intercourse. However, adolescents with the heaviest sexual experience reported watching the most television (Brown, Childers, & Waszak, 1990). This effect was strongest for boys who watched television apart from their parents and who stated that television was their primary source of sexual information. These teens were more likely to believe that premarital and extramarital intercourse with multiple partners were acceptable and were less likely to learn about contraception. In rural areas teens may watch more television due to lack of alternative activities. What is the effect of frequent viewing of rural cable and satellite networks that may provide teens with more sexually explicit material? The answer is unknown but it may be valuable to explore in rural, remote, and frontier communities.

Parental Influence

Adolescents report that they are influenced by their parents' attitudes and behaviors (Humenick et al., 1991). Early sexual experience of the adolescent's mother is associated with an early age of first intercourse in the child, especially girls (Newcomer & Udry, 1985). Boys reporting communication with their mothers regarding sexual matters report a later onset of intercourse. This is not true for communication with fathers, which is associated with greater sexual activity (Hofferth, 1987c). For girls, there was no relation of age of first intercourse with communication with mother or father. The teens' perceptions of their parents' attitudes are often inaccurate (Aneshensel et al., 1990). Parenting education may strengthen parents' skills and effectiveness in communicating their attitudes and beliefs to their children. Education for rural families may necessitate the use of innovative conduits such as town meetings, county extension meetings, and church and school gatherings.

The teens' perceptions of parental disapproval of early sexual intercourse and the physical presence of a supervising adult are associated with a lower rate of sexual activity (Newcomer & Udry, 1985). Adolescents with higher levels of social control in the form of higher attachment to parents, higher commitment to school studies, and more involvement in structured community activities are less likely to initiate early sexual intercourse (Jessor et al., 1983). Indirect "parental" control by a community could be present in the form of supervised alternative activities available to teens. Thus far no studies of the role of the availability of alternative activities have been done.

Peers and Dating

Peers are believed to play a major role in the adolescent's choice to begin or to delay sexual intercourse. Several studies suggest that it is not really peer attitudes and actions that determine an adolescent's actions but rather the teens' perceptions of their peers' activities and beliefs (Humenick et al., 1991). High school students who were asked to describe their peers' beliefs and sexual experience were incorrect almost one half of the time. They were able to predict the beliefs of casual acquaintances with almost the same accuracy as the beliefs of their best friends (Hofferth, 1987c). Honest discussions with peers may be an activity that rural health professionals can facilitate.

Not surprisingly, the age of first intercourse is related to the age of the first date. However, 50% of males said that their first intercourse was outside a dating relationship (Zelnik & Shah, 1983). White adolescents reported a progression from dating to petting to intercourse. Black adolescents reported that intercourse often came before petting or even dating in a relationship (Smith & Udry, 1985). In smaller homogeneous communities it may be possible to influence the "normal" age at which dating begins and the "normal" pattern of dates, that is, group dating, double dating, alcohol-free dating, and other activities available for dating couples.

Personality and Self-Esteem

The teen personality is a critical factor in the initiation of sexual activity. One of the few studies of rural adolescents (Jessor et al., 1983) presents a composite picture of the adolescent most likely to engage in early and frequent sexual activity. This teen places a high value on independence; places a lower value on and has a lower expectation for academic achievement; is more tolerant of socially deviant behavior; is less religious; perceives less compatibility between parents and peers; receives less parental influence compared to the influence of peers; receives more social approval for problem behaviors; displays more problem behaviors; and has lower measured intelligence and academic achievement.

Although many studies have examined the issue of self-esteem, only Orr, Wilbrandt, Brack, Rauch, and Ingersoll (1989) were able to show an association with lower self-esteem in sexually active seventh, eighth, and ninth grade girls. No interaction between sexual activity and self-esteem was seen in boys. However, teens who have higher self-esteem are more likely to use contraception if they are sexually active (Hofferth, 1987a).

Risks, Benefits, and Societal Trends

At least one study has shown an association between the level of sexual activity and the perceived risk/benefit ratio of intercourse during adolescence. Black males express the least perception of risk and the greatest perception of benefit compared to white males and to females of both races (Cvetkovich & Grote, 1980). Meaningful educational experiences of risks and benefits may influence teens' decision making (Paperny & Starn, 1989; Stout & Rivara, 1989). The care of an "egg" or "plant" baby for a week has been used as an educational experience to emphasize the risks of teen pregnancy.

There has been some decline in the overall rate of sexual activity in teens. The decline is less marked for rural than for urban adolescents and for whites than for blacks (Aneshensel et al., 1990). Several factors may be responsible for this change. There is now a decreased ratio of teens to adults, making supervision more likely and more frequent. A religious revival has appeared, particularly in fundamentalist churches and among the baby boom generation. There may also be a ceiling effect: the portion of sexually active teens was never expected to reach 100%. Finally, the fear of AIDS and sexually transmitted diseases may have put a damper on teen sexual activity.

Prevention of Teen Pregnancy

The number of programs introduced nationally to deal with teen pregnancy continues to escalate. Current programs can be based in schools, churches, girls' clubs, YMCAs, scouting troops, or other gatherings of youth. Many communities reach the largest number of children when programs are school-based with the cooperation of other interested groups. Programs directed at delaying the onset of sexual activity focus on the parents, the children, or the parent-child unit. They deal with most of the potentially modifiable factors that are known to affect the initiation of sexual activity and increased contraceptive use.

Achievable goals of teen pregnancy prevention programs can include broader socialization opportunities, career opportunity sessions, and programs to enhance self-esteem and religious affiliation. The family unit can be involved in parent-child communication programs and sessions for parents regarding sex education of children. Teens may organize peer support groups for abstinence and classes on decision-making skills.

Although a few programs have proven effective in one area or another, some do not appear to be effective and most have not been evaluated. A sample of programs that have been sufficiently evaluated to suggest at least some efficacy will be presented here. Meager information about teen pregnancy programs in rural populations is available. Consequently, it is imperative that programs be adopted only after their application to the rural situation and their practical potential for use in the rural community are assessed.

Abstinence Programs

Promotion of abstinence is the goal of at least four programs reported in the literature. Aimed at prevention of sexual activity but using very different methods, each program is planning an evaluation.

Education of adolescents about self-discipline and responsibility in human sexuality is the goal of Emory University's program. Based on four workshops, it is being tested in Atlanta and Cleveland and has shown that participants delay initiation of sexual intercourse for 5 months compared to nonparticipants (Hofferth, 1987b). Now commercially available, it is being used in several rural sites but no data on its efficacy in these populations has been or is being collected. Another project based in Bozeman, Montana, hopes to improve parent-child communication to prevent teen sexual intercourse. The parents help their children develop a better self-image and decision-making skills (Hofferth, 1987b).

A mass media campaign in southern California was successful in increasing the number of reported parent-child conversations regarding sexual matters. The number of parents who stated that they had primary responsibility for their children's sex education also increased minimally. Television was found to be the most effective media resource. No data on the effect of increased parent-child communication on adolescent sexual behavior was collected (Hofferth, 1987b).

The fourth demonstration project presents a value-based curriculum to parents and children through church, school, and community programs. Source, Inc., has measured the information retention in the Values and Choices curriculum to be greater than 80% at 3- and 6-month follow-up (Williams & Bryant, 1989).

School Programs

Studies of schools providing sex education show that such education does increase the students' knowledge about the subject (Yawn & Yawn, 1988). Results of studies differ in their assessments of the impact of education on behavior. All agree that school sex education courses do not result in earlier or increased frequency of intercourse (Zelnik & Kim, 1982). Some studies have reported increased contraceptive use among students receiving sex education in school, whereas others have found none (Stout & Rivara, 1989).

Comprehensive school-based clinics provide all the basics of adolescent health care including care for minor illnesses; athletic, employment, and college physicals; immunizations; weight control programs; and sexual health care. The oldest school-based clinic began in St. Paul, Minnesota, in 1973. Students of the St. Paul schools where these clinics are located showed a decline in birth rates from 59 per thousand in 1976-1977 to 26 per thousand in 1983-1984, whereas national birth rates for both 1977 and 1982 were 45 per thousand adolescents. Whether this decline represents prevention of pregnancies or an increase in pregnancy terminations is unknown (Hofferth, 1987b).

In Baltimore a cooperative effort of Johns Hopkins University and a junior high, a high school, and a nearby freestanding clinic is called the Self Center. Girls who participated in the full 3 years of the program had a 30.1% decrease in pregnancy rates, but the rate in the surrounding control schools increased by 57.6%. A 7-month delay in initiation of sexual intercourse (especially among junior high students) and increases in clinic and contraceptive use were recorded. Younger students, particularly junior high boys, showed a substantial use of the center's services (Hardy, 1987).

A unique aspect of some school programs is the use of interactive computer programs. One program developed in New Orleans (Paperny & Starn, 1989) allows students to rehearse decision-making skills, and another program called "The Baby Game" explores alternatives and consequences of sexual activity (Alemi, Cherry, & Meffert, 1989). Both programs increase knowledge but neither has been assessed as a method to modify behavior.

Community-Based Programs

A broad-based educational program aimed at the reduction of adolescent pregnancy has been reported in a rural South Carolina community. The program included evaluation of local problems; education of school, church, health professionals, and lay adults in the community; and a coordinated school and church curriculum in kindergarten through twelfth grades. The program showed a decline in pregnancy rates of 59% in the 14- to 17-year-olds after 3 years. Surrounding communities recorded a 25.3% increase in the pregnancy rate during this same period (Vincent, Clearie, & Schluchter, 1987).

Several large urban hospitals have become involved in teen pregnancy prevention. Some hospitals provide special hospital-based adolescent health clinics, whereas others provide staff for school-based health clinics. Most of these hospitals also provide education support to the area's junior and senior high schools.

Male-Only Programs

Several rural counties of Virginia have developed programs to target rural black males (Watson & Kelly, 1990). After several attempts to develop support groups, they began to provide a series of ten 90-minute sessions for any males between the ages 12 to 18 who agreed to attend. The topics to be covered in these sessions are determined by the group in attendance. The discussions are facilitated by nursing, social work, and medical students and staff from the South Hampton Road AHEC, a rural Virginia Area Health Education Center that provides rural experiences to health profession students. Although evaluation of the program is only beginning, the increasing class size, and the pre- and posttest knowledge test scores suggest that this is a successful program aimed at the often ignored or forgotten at-risk male (Meyer, 1991). The program directors comment that a snack or picnic supper seems to improve attendance.

Recommendations and Conclusions

Many teen pregnancy prevention programs have been developed around the country, but not many have been assessed thoroughly, even in urban communities. One cannot simply copy an existing program and expect it to be effective in a rural area. Extensive reference material and detailed guidelines for implementing sexuality education programs are readily available (Cook, Kirby, Wilson, & Alter, 1984; Planned Parenthood, 1990).

Developing a program for a rural area should begin with an effort to overcome the ever-present denial that a problem exists. The population at risk should be characterized in terms of race, socioeconomic status, and other factors relevant to the initiation of sexual intercourse, so that the timing of the intervention and targeting of the groups at highest risk can be planned.

In each community energetic and knowledgeable facilitators and leaders are required to organize and to spearhead the project. The nurse, physician, or social worker who has a background in personal and public health, the psychosocial attributes of health problems, and communication and integration skills is often the most appropriate community leader. School health nurses have an obvious role, but office and hospital nurses can provide information and support to teens in their occupational facilities. In rural communities physicians are often asked by neighbors, friends, relatives, churches, and schools for advice and education. Viewed as leaders and respected for their education and dedication, rural physicians can and must be at least coleaders in these important efforts.

Finally, parents, schools, churches, and any available, interested community groups must be involved in any teen pregnancy prevention program at the outset. The use of the media, especially television, is advantageous. A convenient family planning clinic is optimal. The program must also address other teen health risks, including the use of alcohol, tobacco, and drugs, and the risks of sexually transmitted diseases. The common rural problems of isolation, increased time and distance for travel, and lack of confidentiality and anonymity require unique local solutions.

References

Alemi, F., Cherry, F., & Meffert, G. (1989). Rehearsing decisions may help teenagers: An evaluation of a simulation game. *Computers & Biology in Medicine, 19*(4), 283-290.

Aneshensel, C. S., Becerra, R. M., Fielder, E. P., & Schuler, R. H. (1990). Onset of fertility-related events during adolescence: A prospective comparison of Mexican American and non-Hispanic white females. *American Journal of Public Health, 80*(8), 959-963.

Billy, J. O. G., Rodgers, J. L., & Udry, J. R. (1984). Adolescent sexual behavior and friendship choice. *Social Forces, 62*, 653-678.

Blum, R. W. (1988). The Minnesota Adolescent Health Survey: Implications for physicians. *Minnesota Medicine, 71,* 143-145.

Brown, J. D., Childers, K. W., & Waszak, C. S. (1990). Television and adolescent sexuality. *Journal of Adolescent Health Care, 11*(10), 52-57.

Cook, A. T., Kirby, D., Wilson, P., & Alter, J. (1984). *Sexuality education: A guide to developing and implementing programs.* Santa Cruz, CA: Network Publications.

Cvetkovich, G., & Grote, B. (1980). Psychosocial development and the social problem of teenage illegitimacy. In C. Chilman (Ed.), *Adolescent pregnancy and childbearing* (pp. 15-41). Washington, DC: Government Printing Office.

Donovan, C. (1990). Adolescent sexuality. *British Medical Journal 300*(6731), 1026-1027.

Ensminger, M. E. (1987). Adolescent sexual behavior as it relates to other transition behaviors in youth. In S. L. Hofferth & C. D. Hayes (Eds.), *Risking the future* (pp. 36-55). Washington, DC: National Academy Press.

Hardy, J. B. (1987, July). Preventing adolescent pregnancy: Counseling teens and their parents. *Medical Aspects of Human Sexuality,* pp. 32-38.

Hayes, C. D. (1987). Adolescent pregnancy and childbearing: An emerging research focus. In S. L. Hofferth & C. D. Hayes (Eds.), *Risking the future* (pp. 1-6). Washington, DC: National Academy Press.

Hofferth, S. L. (1987a). Contraceptive decision-making among adolescents. In S. L. Hofferth & C. D. Hayes (Eds.), *Risking the future* (pp. 56-77). Washington, DC: National Academy Press.

Hofferth, S. L. (1987b). The effect of programs and policies on adolescent pregnancy and childbearing. In S. L. Hofferth & C. D. Hayes (Eds.), *Risking the future,* (pp. 207-263). Washington, DC: National Academy Press.

Hofferth, S. L. (1987c). Influences on early sexual and fertility behavior. In S. L. Hofferth & C. D. Hayes (Eds.), *Risking the future* (pp. 7-35). Washington, DC: National Academy Press.

Humenick, S. S., Wilkerson, N. N., & Paul, N. W. (Eds.). (1991). Adolescent pregnancy: Nursing prospectus on prevention. *Birth Defects, 27*(1), 1-275.

Jessor, R., Costa, F., Jessor, S. L., & Donovan, J. E. (1983). Time of first intercourse: A prospective study. *Journal of Personality and Social Psychology, 44,* 608-626.

McAnarney E. R., & Hendee, W. R. (1989a). Adolescent pregnancy and its consequences. *Journal of the American Medical Association, 262,* 74-77.

McAnarney, E. R., & Hendee, W. R. (1989b). The prevention of adolescent pregnancy. *Journal of the American Medical Association, 262,* 78-82.

Meyer, V. F. (1991). A critique of adolescent pregnancy prevention research: The invisible white male. *Adolescence, 26*(101), 217-222.

Newcomer, S. F., & Udry, J. R. (1985). Parent-child communication and adolescent sexual behavior. *Family Planning Perspectives, 17,* 169-174.

Orr, D. P., Wilbrandt, M. L., Brack, C. J., Rauch, S. P., & Ingersoll, G. M. (1989). Reported sexual behaviors and self-esteem among young adolescents. *American Journal of Diseases of Children, 143*(1), 86-90.

Paperny, D. M., & Starn, J. R. (1989). Adolescent pregnancy prevention by health education computer games: Computer-assisted instruction of knowledge and attitudes. *Pediatrics, 83*(5), 742-752.

Planned Parenthood Federation of America, Inc. (1990). *First things first: A planned parenthood initiative to reduce adolescent childbearing by 50 percent by 1999.* New York: Author.

Raines, T. G. (1991). Family-focused primary prevention of adolescent pregnancy. *Birth Defects, 27*(1), 87-103.

Smith, E. A., & Udry, J. R. (1985). Coital and non-coital sexual behaviors of white and black adolescents. *American Journal of Public Health, 75,* 1200-1203.

Stout, J. W., & Rivara, F. P. (1989). Schools and sex education: Does it work? *Pediatrics, 83*(3), 375-379.

Swenson, I., Erickson, D., Ehlinger, E., Carlson, G., & Swaney, S. (1989). Fertility, menstrual characteristics, and contraceptive practices among white, black, and Southeast Asian refugee adolescents. *Adolescence, 24*(95), 647-654.

Udry, J. R., Billy, J. O. G., Morris, N. M., Groff, T. R., & Raj, M. H. (1985). Serum androgenic hormones motivate sexual behavior in adolescent boys. *Fertility and Sterility, 43,* 90-94.

Udry, J. R., Talbert, R., & Morris, M. N. (1986). Biosocial foundations for adolescent female sexuality. *Demography, 23,* 217-230.

Vincent, M. L., Clearie, A. F., & Schluchter, M. D. (1987). Reducing adolescent pregnancy through school and community-based education. *Journal of the American Medical Association 257,* 3382-3386.

Watson, F. I., & Kelly, M. J. (1990). Targeting the at-risk male: A strategy for adolescent pregnancy prevention. *Journal of the National Medical Association, 81,* 453-456.

Williams, D. L., & Bryant, N. (1989). What influences teenagers' decisions about sex? *Source, 4,* 1-3. [Newsletter for Search Institute, Inc., Minneapolis, MN]

Yawn, B. P., & Yawn, R. A. (1987). Teenage sexual activity in rural Minnesota. *Minnesota Medicine, 70,* 38-39.

Yawn, B. P., & Yawn, R. A. (1988). Teen age sexuality education in rural Minnesota. *Minnesota Medicine, 71,* 147-149.

Zelnik, M., & Kantner, J. (1980). Sexual activity, contraceptive use and pregnancy among metropolitan-area teenagers. *Family Planning Perspectives, 12,* 230-237.

Zelnik, M., Kantner, J., & Ford, K. (1981). *Sex and pregnancy in adolescence.* Beverly Hills, CA: Sage.

Zelnik, M., & Kim, Y. J. (1982). Sex education and its association with teenage sexual activity, pregnancy and contraceptive use. *Family Planning Perspectives, 14,* 117-126.

Zelnik, M., & Shah, F. K. (1983). First intercourse among young Americans. *Family Planning Perspectives, 15,* 64-70.

8
■ ■ ■

Common Mental Health Problems

LAWRENCE P. PETERSON

Introduction

The greatest concentration of psychiatrists remains, as it has always been, in larger urban areas. The phasing out of the large, often rural state psychiatric hospitals in the 1960s and the 1970s not only placed many of the chronically mentally ill in communities that were not prepared to take care of them but also moved even more mental health professionals into urban settings.

This is ironic in that it has happened in conjunction with a relative renaissance in the field of psychiatry itself. There has been a more rapid increase in the understanding of neurophysiology and functional neuroanatomy than at any previous point in the history of medicine. Both basic research and techniques in the area of brain imaging are radically transforming some of our most deeply held theories of human behavior. This has led to significant advances in treatment; and where emotional support was once the only thing a physician could offer, there are now virtual cures. These changes have inevitably led to confusion with introduction of several new medications a year and seemingly unending changes in terminology.

Because of both the uneven distribution of psychiatrists and the common occurrence of emotional disorders, the rural practitioner has always been and will continue to be a primary dispenser of mental health services. In this chapter we will consider several of the most common mental health problems and the means to identify and treat them. These problems include the depression and anxiety disorders, now seen as biochemical relatives of one another and often sharing the same treatment approaches; the functional psychoses, as in the schizophrenic disorders and bipolar disorders or psychoses as complications of Alzheimer's disease or stroke; and finally, one of the most frustrating areas of any practice, chemical dependency and its impact both physiologically and socially on the patient and his family.

Up to one half of the patients that come into a rural family practice clinic may be there because of primary psychiatric disorders. These individuals also tend to take up more time than the purely medical cases. The local mental health center, if one is available, may provide help but just as often they may refer the patient back to you asking for help with medications because they have no psychiatric coverage. These patients may be among the most grateful in your practice because of the potentially dramatic improvement they experience. It is important to see disorders like depression as very debilitating conditions over which the patient has little control. The manifestations of depression may be colored by the patient's unique personality style, life experiences, intelligence, and ethnic and social background. These same factors that complicate the diagnosis and treatment of emotional disorders can also make illnesses such as diabetes or hypertension difficult to manage. One of the things that attracts many to medicine is the challenge of the puzzle that the patient presents, and the psychiatric disorders are some of the most fascinating mysteries in medicine. When seen as a manageable challenge this aspect of a practice can be very satisfying.

The Mood Disorders

The mood or affective disorders represent the most common psychiatric problems requiring physician intervention, occurring in 4% to 6% of the population. The overwhelming majority of these patients who seek medical attention can and are treated by nonpsychiatric professionals, but at least 50% are never treated at all. This occurs in spite of the enormous suffering that these individuals endure. Many of us would choose to have any other disease over a mood disorder; and about 15% of major depressive disorder patients choose death by suicide. The diagnosis crosses all socioeconomic lines and is fairly consistent in frequency from culture to culture. About twice as many women are diagnosed as men, though this may be significantly biased by the differences in the willingness to ask for help. Children and adolescents are almost as frequently depressed as adults with the overall incidence dropping off in the elderly.

Definitions

There are several different disorders traveling under the common label of depression. These include major depressive disorder, dysthymic disorder, uncomplicated or prolonged grief, and adjustment disorder with depression. The manic depressive or bipolar disorders will be considered in the next section. The focus in this section will be on the major depressive disorders. These are defined by the American Psychiatric Association's diagnostic manual as a change in functioning of at least 2 weeks' duration characterized by a depressed mood or a lack of interest or pleasure that must be accompanied by several of the following:

- weight loss or gain
- insomnia or hypersomnia
- psychomotor agitation or retardation
- fatigue
- feelings of worthlessness
- guilt
- decreased concentration
- thoughts of death or suicide

The disorder may occur as a single episode or in a recurrent pattern, such as seasonally. The dysthymic disorders encompass the old concept of depressive neurosis, with a depressed mood for most of the day occurring over a 2-year period, without clear symptoms of a major depressive episode. Grief or uncomplicated bereavement is the normal reaction to significant loss and may appear very similar to a major depressive episode, but it is time limited and clearly related to events. The adjustment disorders with depressed mood are essentially overreactions to events with a sad mood that may last no more than 6 months.

Evaluation

The core of any evaluation is a complete history with appropriate questions regarding the symptoms of depression, particularly in regard to sleep patterns, loss of energy, suicide, any previous treatment and family history. In men it is valuable to ask about irritability, which may occur more frequently than sadness. Major depression has a significant genetic component and one should ask about any relatives with a history of depression, anxiety, or suicide. The Beck Depression Inventory is a short, effective way of assessing the presence and depth of a depression. The Minnesota Multiphasic Personality Inventory (MMPI) is a very sensitive self-administered test that must be sent away for computer scoring. It is returned with an extensive narrative that may help in the diagnosis of a variety of conditions and mixed disorders.

Early dementias and small stroke syndrome should be ruled out and the patient's current medications should be reviewed. Medications that may cause depression include antihypertensives, oral contraceptives, steroids, cimetidine, hypnotics, tranquilizers, beta-blockers, and stimulants. Alcoholism must also be routinely ruled out. A physical examination and laboratory evaluation including thyroid testing should be done.

Treatment

For the grief states and some of the adjustment disorders, brief supportive counseling in the exam room may be of great help. More severe depressive disorders should involve a psychotherapist. Data generally show that the best recovery rates for major depressive disorders occur when there is the concomitant use of antidepressant medication and talking therapy. Currently, a form called Cognitive Therapy has shown the most promise in the treatment of depression. This approach assumes that depressed persons automatically make a variety of depressogenic assumptions about themselves and their environment that can be slowly pointed out and corrected. Often the therapist will want to work with a physician in the use of medications.

Antidepressant medications have been available for more than 30 years and are the backbone of the treatment for major depressive disorders. These medications may be divided into monoamine oxidase inhibitors, tricyclics, heterocyclics, and new or third-generation agents. Most of the new agents fall into the class of selective serotonin reuptake inhibitors of which fluoxetine (Prozac) is a prime example. The monoamine oxidase inhibitors are not useful in the

Table 8.1 Commonly Used Antidepressants and Doses

Class	Name	Dosage Range (mg)
Tricyclics		
	Imipramine (Tofranil)	75-300
	Desipramine (Norpramin)	75-150
	Amitriptyline (Elavil)	75-300
	Nortriptyline (Pamelor)	75-150
	Doxepin (Sinequan)	75-300
	Trimipramine (Surmontil)	75-300
	Protriptyline (Vivactil)	15-60
Second Generation		
	Maprotiline (Ludiomil)	75-250
	Amoxapine (Asendin)	75-300
	Trazadone (Desyrel)	150-300
Third Generation (Selective Serotonin Reuptake Inhibitors)		
	Clomipramine (Anafranil)*	75-250
	Fluoxetine (Prozac)	20-80
	Sertraline (Zoloft)	50-200
Third Generation (Nonserotonin)		
	Bupropion (Wellbutrin)	200-350

NOTE: *Anafranil is licensed only as a treatment for obsessive compulsive disorder.

general practice of medicine and there is a rapidly developing preference for the newer generation medications.

All of these compounds are equally effective but do not work equally well for each patient. The primary differences are in side effects, with the older compounds having prominent antihistaminic and anticholinergic effects and the newer antidepressants having serotonergic effects (nausea and agitation). All take up to 2 weeks to work and doses should be slowly advanced. Table 8.1 lists examples of first-, second-, and third-generation antidepressants and their commonly effective doses. The period of use is generally 6 months to a year, after which time the dose should be tapered off to avoid the mild withdrawal effects and to allow the patient to see how lower doses are tolerated before testing the ability to be undepressed without medication. The tricyclic compounds have a moderate effect on cardiac conduction and a significant postural hypotensive effect that must be kept in mind in the elderly. It is good for the family physician to develop a familiarity with two or three anti-depressants while realizing that one or more new drugs may be introduced each year. Each physician should be familiar with a tricyclic and a selective serotonin reuptake inhibitor.

There are several other organic therapies available for the treatment of depression. Electroconvulsive therapy remains an effective treatment that is of value in patients who cannot tolerate medications or who are in an acute depressive crisis where risk for self-harm or dangerous and overt neglect is obvious. Patients with seasonal affective disorder (SAD) are extremely sensitive to ambient light levels and are prone to develop depression in the fall and winter. These patients may respond to short periods of exposure to high-intensity lights on a daily basis. Most medical supply houses will rent photo-therapy lights for a winter season. Exercise has been clearly shown to benefit most depressed patients and a daily schedule of a sustained cardiovascular workout will be a useful adjunct to medications or talking therapy.

Referral

The primary reason for referral of patients with depressive disorders is unresponsiveness to treatment, most often due to doses of antidepressants that are too low for the given patient or inadequate length of use. When there is a failure to respond to trials of at least two medications at adequate doses, a referral to a psychiatrist should be entertained. There are a number of possible complications in mood disorders that usually necessitate consultation. Some of these are coexisting severe personality disorders such as borderline syndromes, a history of sexual abuse, dementia, and unusual or idiosyncratic antidepressant medication effects. Repeated cycles of depression after successful treatment are another reason for referral. Suicidal threats should always be taken seriously, even in the person with a history of suicidal gestures. The burden of being the only helping person working with a suicidal patient is great and should be shared by involving a psychotherapist, referral to a psychiatrist, or, in acute situations, hospitalization. It must always be remembered that depression is a potentially fatal disease and that even after the best efforts of all involved, a patient may take his or her life.

Prevention

The education of the community and your own patient population is the main preventive step a family physician can take. Excellent materials are available from a variety of sources including the National Institute of Mental Health, the American Psychiatric Association and the American Psychiatric Press, and the Dean Foundation. Materials covering depression and anxiety disorders quickly disappear when placed in waiting rooms and prompt more informed patient questions. Families with a history of affective disorders should be encouraged to share the family history with their own children and relatives both to reduce stigma and to give permission to others to ask for help. Those with a family history of depression may benefit from attempts to reduce life stress, to exercise, and to order one's life. Stable home situations and a strong belief system are both helpful preventives and make the treatment of an existing depression easier.

Anxiety Disorders

The anxiety disorders represent the most common of the psychiatric syndromes. They often masquerade as other medical or psychiatric conditions. There have been significant changes in the treatment of these conditions over the past few years, reflecting the understanding that they have a lot in common with the mood disorders. Up to 20% of the population have one or another of the phobias, and as many as 10% of primary care patients have panic symptoms. The incidence of obsessive-compulsive disorders is constantly being revised upward and it is difficult even to estimate the numbers of anxious somaticizing patients that make repeated visits to the doctor's office. Anxiety problems also appear when the threat of serious medical illness is present; an ill patient may lead to an anxious family member. These disorders may be present at all ages with women more commonly represented than men.

Definitions

The difficulties in dealing with the anxiety disorders start immediately with the definition and the discussion of the syndrome.

Whether in the office or the graduate school classroom, these are not easy problems to describe despite their universal nature. Anxiety is basically a physiologic fear response with an inadequate stimulus, an excessive duration, or a paralyzing effect on behavior. There is motor tension, autonomic hyperactivity, and vigilance or scanning. A generalized anxiety disorder is a chronic state of anxiety with the individual worrying about two or more life situations. A phobic disorder is excessive anxiety triggered by a specific stimulus that results in avoidant behavior. Panic disorder is a discrete period of intense fear that is not clearly related to a specific stimulus and is accompanied by any number of symptoms that include tachycardia, hyperventilation, nausea, and a fear of dying or going crazy. Panic disorder often mimics cardiac or respiratory conditions. Agoraphobia is a fear of crowds or situations that would be uncomfortable in the event of a panic attack. This disorder often confines people to their homes, making it impossible for them to obtain help. There are a variety of other anxiety-related syndromes such as obsessive-compulsive disorder in which the sufferer is paralyzed by recurrent intrusive thoughts or ritualistic behaviors—cleaning and checking, for example. There is a large group of somatiform disorders characterized by a preoccupation with physical symptoms or worry about illness. These disorders become wrapped around legitimate organic diseases and create endless problems in diagnosis and management.

Evaluation

In obtaining a history the doctor must ask about the condition in several ways. Words like *nervous, worry, tension, stress, fear, panic, hypertension, agitated,* and *"about to have a nervous breakdown"* may all be synonymous with what we refer to as anxiety. The duration and stimulus for these symptoms should be elicited and the family history scanned for anyone with either nervous or depressive disorders. Suicide should be asked about because some of these patients are at significant risk even in the absence of depression. Symptoms of a major depression may coexist with an anxiety problem and can alert the doctor to a more severe problem than a little nervousness. The MMPI is a good test with a variety of scales for picking up anxiety disorders. But a good history remains the most effective screening device.

Anxiety may present as a physical disorder and vice versa, so a complete physical examination and appropriate laboratory studies are essential. The list of look-a-like conditions is long but generally consists of cardiac disease with rhythm disturbances; endocrinological problems, particularly of the thyroid; neurological diseases such as demyelinating conditions or vertigo; and drug or medication effects. One of the most common iatrogenic causes of anxiety is excess caffeine intake.

Thyroid studies, an electrocardiogram, pulmonary function testing, and serum glucose should be performed.

Treatment

The acute treatment of anxiety disorders remains much the same as it has been for the past 20 years, with benzodiazepines as the preferred medication. These medications are very effective, have a generally low level of sedation, interact negatively with few medications, and have a very low toxicity. Although tolerance quickly develops to sedative and euphoric effects, it is now known that the antianxiety effect goes on indefinitely. These medications are indicated for the control of acute anxiety and for initiating treatment in panic disorders while longer term treatment can be instituted. The more intermediate acting medications are preferable. Benzodiazepines should not be used for more than 6 weeks except in cases of severe disorders. It is best to obtain an outside opinion before writing any prescriptions for chronic benzodiazepine use.

Recently, antidepressants have come into widespread use for the treatment of panic disorder and chronic or generalized anxiety. Selective serotonin reuptake blockers such as Prozac are now being used for the treatment of obsessional anxiety. The dosages range more widely than when treating depression, so smaller amounts are worth trying initially. Virtually all of the tricyclics and new generation antidepressants work for this purpose. The beta-blockers have enjoyed some success in the treatment of panic disorder and social anxiety but may reduce physical symptoms while leaving the subjective sense of fear untouched. This produces a very unsettled feeling in some patients. A newer nonbenzodiazepine (buspirone or Buspar) has shown some success with obsessional anxiety and general anxiety. There is no withdrawal or risk of abuse, but buspirone must be used regularly and it takes several days to weeks to become effective. There has been some promising research in the use of anticonvulsants in the treatment of panic disorder, but their use remains experimental.

Cognitive and behavior psychotherapies have been very success-ful, particularly in the treatment of phobias and panic disorder, and are indicated in all anxiety disorders. It is wise to have a good working relationship with a therapist familiar with these techniques. This kind of working relationship is very valuable with the anxious, somaticizing patient who can benefit from seeing a single primary physician regularly to manage any medicines and a therapist (psy-chologist or psychiatrist) who can do cognitive behavioral work with the anxiety. As with the mood disorders, exercise is beneficial, though the anxious patient is often difficult to motivate because of a fear that exercise will worsen the condition.

Referral

The majority of anxiety disorders are probably treatable in the primary care office, and the chief reason for referral is lack of ade-quate control of symptoms. The second most common reason is for another opinion about long-term benzodiazepine use or concern about dependency. Any patient who comes into the office and re-quests these medications by generic name should arouse suspicion. Severe or frequently occurring panic disorders and obsessive com-pulsive disorders should be referred for an initial evaluation; the anxiety disorder patient with suicidal ideation merits an immediate psychiatric evaluation. After consultation and some initial medica-tion management or therapy a majority of patients can be referred back to the primary care doctor.

Prevention

Prevention of the anxiety disorders is much the some as with the depressive disorders and centers on education that will encourage more patients to come forward for treatment. No group is more unwilling to initiate a request for help than people with anxiety disorders, who often feel that they are the only ones to suffer from this problem. The irony is that very effective treatments are avail-able if doctor and patient are willing to work together.

Psychotic Disorders

The primary psychotic disorders are the schizophrenias, a spectrum of diseases. The risk of developing schizophrenia over a lifetime is about 1%. These disorders begin in late adolescence or young adulthood and usually last indefinitely. They are extremely debilitating and discouraging to the patient and family. The manic depressive or bipolar disorders occur less frequently and are more appropriately classified with the mood disorders, but they are included here because the acute manic phase of the cycle often appears indistinguishable from a schizophrenic episode.

Definitions

The Diagnostic and Statistical Manual of the American Psychiatric Association defines schizophrenia as a disorder with a set of psychotic symptoms such as delusions, hallucinations, loosening of associations, or grossly inappropriate behavior that substantially interferes with the person's life and has been present for at least 6 months. There are several phases of these diseases, and many types of schizophrenia are diagnosed on the basis of an array of symptoms.

Kurt Schneider lists a series of "first rank" symptoms for schizophrenia that are helpful in making a diagnosis. These are:

- hearing one's thoughts aloud
- auditory hallucinations that comment on one's behavior
- somatic hallucinations
- feeling one's thoughts are controlled
- the spreading of thoughts to others
- delusions

There are also second rank symptoms that include mood disturbance and a flat affect.

A manic episode occurring as part of a bipolar disorder is characterized by episode of elevated or irritable mood with grandiosity that causes an impairment in overall functioning. Paranoia, delusional thinking, and occasional hallucinations can occur in mania and make the diagnosis easily confused with the schizophreniform

disorders. Complicating these disorders are brief reactive psychoses that may occur as single episodes and drug-related psychoses,
both of which may be symptomatically indistinguishable from the
major disorders except by history. Certain personality disorders
such as schizoid or schizotypal personality may be difficult to separate from the chronic and insidiously developing psychoses. The
dementias from Parkinson's disease, Alzheimer's disease, and multiple small strokes may present as a psychotic management problems, but are usually identifiable by the age of onset.

Evaluation

The primary care doctor is often the first professional consulted
when a psychotic episode occurs. A good history, usually obtained
from friends or family, may help rule out iatrogenic causes. A family
history is common in bipolar disorders (particularly a history of
suicide or alcohol abuse) and less common or nonexistent in schizophrenia. The physical examination and history may help rule out
organic causes such as an encephalopathy (Huntington's or Wilson's disease), seizure disorder, thyroid dysfunction, and drug toxicity that may include over-the-counter medication abuse. Serum
electrolytes, blood glucose, thyroid studies, calcium levels, liver
functions, hemogram, and a urine drug screen are all helpful. In the
more protracted psychoses psychological testing in the form of an
MMPI or a Rorschach test may uncover more seriously disordered
thinking.

Treatment

The first goal of treatment is to provide a secure environment,
and this may be accomplished initially in a general hospital. Whether
inpatient or outpatient treatment is elected, the medications of choice
are the major tranquilizers. These medications are more appropriately thought of as chemical restraints rather than tranquilizing
medications, and have a variety of fairly significant side effects such
as Parkinsonian symptoms, motor agitation, sexual dysfunction,
heat intolerance, blunted affect, and the long-term, irreversible condition called tardive dyskinesia. Practitioners should be familiar
with the presentation of these side effects. The high potency, low

dose neuroleptics are preferred, such as haloperidol (Haldol) and trifluoperazine (Stelazine).

In an acute situation these medications should be given intramuscularly if the patient will not take them orally or if the situation is urgent. The bipolar patient is often stabilized with neuroleptics before lithium therapy is begun. The initiation of lithium should be done by a psychiatrist familiar with the peculiarities of this drug.

In the psychotic dementia of the elderly, neuroleptics should be started at the smallest possible daily dose and advanced slowly while side effects are carefully watched. For example, haloperidol may be used at doses of 0.5 to 1.0 milligrams daily and advanced every 3 to 4 days. The reasons for the medication and attempts at withdrawal in the first few months should be clearly documented. The same suggestions apply in the use of these medicines with the developmentally disabled. In all cases adjunct therapy for side effects (Cogentin, Artane, Benadryl, Symmetrel) should not be used unless side effects actually appear. After several weeks, attempts should be made to reduce side effect medications.

Attempts to control the symptoms of the chronically mentally ill patient with medication must be tempered with the realization that community-based programs (mental health centers, day treatment, and sheltered workshops) are critical to preventing relapse and for providing a quality existence for the patient. Treatment of these people is always a partnership.

Referral

Virtually all schizophrenic and bipolar patients should be referred for a complete diagnostic evaluation. The psychoses secondary to iatrogenic causes or dementing illnesses are largely treated by the primary care physician. Consultation is obviously desirable when the response to treatment is inadequate but may also be required by some state regulatory agencies when the patient is in a facility like a nursing home. A psychiatrist may be involved if the patient needs involuntary commitment for treatment. Because the neuroleptic drugs can produce such a range of side effects, periodic consultation for the purpose of reviewing medications may be advisable.

Prevention

Unfortunately we know so little about the schizophrenias and the etiology of the psychoses that prevention is not a realistic concept. As with the other disorders, education is an undertaking within the scope of the rural physician by providing information that demythologizes mental illness.

Chemical Dependency

Chemical dependency is one of the most common and universally hidden problems in a medical practice. Various estimates place a 120 billion dollar cost on the effects of chemical use. One half of suicides, one half of fatal car accidents, one quarter of all hospital admissions, and 60% of all violent crimes are directly related to chemical use and abuse. Virtually all chemically dependent people deny the existence of a problem on routine medical examinations, making our normal method of investigation immediately ineffective. Physicians simply must have a high level of suspicion and be aware of red flags, such as the increased incidence of head and neck tumors in alcoholics and unusually difficult to control hypertension. Unfortunately, every mood-altering chemical may have a different "signature" so that the family physician may only be able to detect the more common abuse situations. The primary drug of abuse in rural America is alcohol, but virtually every other substance is readily available. Rural settings may be the preferred distribution sites, processing centers, and growing areas for many illegal drugs.

Definitions

Because of alcohol's availability and social history, alcoholism remains our primary drug-related health problem. When interviewing a suspected alcoholic, a doctor will become embroiled in a debate over definitions. Officially a person is drug dependent when he or she demonstrates a loss of control over drug use; an interference in occupational, social, physical, or emotional functioning; and a tolerance or withdrawal pattern. The following simple definition often works best in clinical situations: "An individual is chemically dependent when drug use interferes with job, family, health, emotions, or legal status and he or she does not alter or cease chemical use over the long run."

This definition also applies to illegal substances or street drugs, with the use being more clandestine. The most common of these is marijuana. At one time it was thought that marijuana did not produce tolerance and dependence but that view is changing, particularly in chronic users. The drug decreases vigilance and attention and produces cognitive impairment that some researchers believe can be permanent. It is also mildly hallucinogenic with panic attacks, paranoid reactions, and hallucinations occurring as unwanted side effects. Most significantly, marijuana is retained in the body's lipid stores where it can exert a continuing effect over months. Cocaine and its derivatives are widely used now, mostly as crack. Cocaine in all of its forms is a potent stimulant and perhaps the most psychologically addicting drug known. It is used intravenously, smoked, and inhaled. There can be significant psychotic episodes and there is no clear physiologic withdrawal. The opiates have been continuously abused in the form of prescription drugs but there has been a renewed use of heroin, often in conjunction with other compounds. The latter is used intravenously and as a consequence is closely associated with the problem of AIDS transmission. Heroin produces tolerance and has a withdrawal—very similar to a gastroenteritis—that is rarely life threatening in severity.

Like heroin, there has been an increase in the use of a variety of hallucinogens including LSD, PCP (phencyclidine), and mushrooms (psilocybin and mescaline). The primary problems with these compounds are panic reactions, delirium, psychoses, and flashbacks. There is no physiologic dependence or withdrawal. The primary prescription drugs of abuse are the narcotics and the remaining barbiturate medicines that are often found in headache preparations. Although the minor tranquilizers are to be closely monitored, the tolerance to the euphoric effects is so rapid that they are less commonly primary drugs of abuse but may be used by the dependent person to enhance the effect or to control withdrawal from other substances.

Table 8.2 The CAGE Questionnaire for Screening for Alcoholism

C- Have you ever felt the need to Cut down on drinking?
A- Have you ever been Annoyed by criticism about your drinking?
G- Have you ever had Guilt feelings about drinking?
E- Have you ever taken a morning Eye opener?

NOTE: A score of two or more positive answers has a sensitivity of 74% and a specificity of 91%.
SOURCES: Buchsbaum et al., 1991; Mayfield et al., 1974.

Evaluation

The most important feature of a chemical dependency workup is a complete history, with attention to patterns of usage. The most commonly neglected question is whether the patient has ever been diagnosed or treated as chemically dependent in the past. It is essential to obtain relevant history from a family member or close friend who may give far more accurate information on chemical use. There are a variety of checklists to administer in an assessment, including the CAGE questionnaire (Table 8.2) and the McAndrews scale on the MMPI. A complete medical examination should be done with attention to findings such as acne rosacea, palmar erythema, nicotine staining, spider angiomas, parotid enlargement, hepatomegaly, signs of peripheral neuropathy, and a level of personal care below what one would expect from the patient. Some of the same findings may occur with chemicals other than alcohol. Laboratory test should include a liver panel (gamma-glutamyl transpeptidase or GGT is elevated in 50% of alcoholic patients), hemogram, glucose, electrolytes, calcium, magnesium, albumin, and prothrombin time.

Treatment

The first goal of treatment is to gain the cooperation of the patient. Although more than 90% of admissions to treatment units are voluntary, meaning no legal commitment, an overwhelming majority of patients are there because of pressure from people such as employers or spouses. Whereas the desire for help is very important in most emotional conditions, in chemical dependency treatment coercion is quite acceptable and does not preclude a successful outcome.

The next issue is handling withdrawal, which in the case of alcohol can rarely be managed successfully as an outpatient. Because of the risk of thiamine deficiency a dose of 100 milligrams intramuscularly or intravenously should be given initially, followed by daily doses of 50 to 100 milligrams. Chlordiazepoxide (Librium) is still the medication of choice for alcohol withdrawal and can be administered in doses of 25 to 50 milligrams orally every 2 hours or less frequently, with a usual maximum daily dose of 400 milligrams. The benzodiazepines are generally absorbed better if given orally than if administered intramuscularly. Slow intravenous administration of diazepam (Valium) may be used in patients who cannot take medication orally. Fluid and electrolyte balance should be monitored, particularly if there is agitation, fever, or fluid loss. The acute withdrawal may take 3 to 5 days.

The help of a trained alcohol counselor is invaluable in pursuing treatment and the patient must be discharged to a suitable inpatient or outpatient treatment program. Successful withdrawal alone is not treatment! The family should be clearly informed that their participation in treatment is essential because this is truly a family disease. The long-term follow-up invariably involves Alcoholics Anonymous as well as possible individual counseling, and support groups such as Alanon, Alateen, and Adult Children of Alcoholics programs. It is very helpful for the rural physician to have attended a local "open" AA meeting to become familiar with the program. Individual programs such as Narcotics Anonymous deal with specialized needs. A list of all the local meetings can be obtained from any Alcoholics Anonymous club and should be part of the informational materials available in the medical office.

The use of Antabuse (disulfiram) is often very helpful, because the decision to drink can be made just once a day or several times a week rather than minute by minute. Monitored Antabuse is usually more successful when a patient has recently completed a treatment program. It can be given in doses of 250 milligrams daily or as little as twice a week. The patient should be in good general health and be free of permanent liver damage. A rare patient may get euphoria from the combination of Antabuse and alcohol.

Referral

Chemical dependency should always be treated by therapists who specialize in drug dependent patients. Some patients merit immediate referral to a psychiatrist or a physician specializing in chemical dependency medicine. These are individuals with histories of multiple relapses, dual diagnosis cases such as people with schizophrenia and alcoholism, and the occasional convoluted legal problems where treatment may be mandated by the courts.

Prevention

The best prevention is education both on a one-to-one level in the office and in increased community awareness. School programs have been shown to decrease and delay adolescent alcohol use and abuse. The children of alcoholics should be encouraged to attend Alateen or Adult Children of Alcoholics classes. It may also be possible to detect the potentially chemically dependent person early by proper questioning and a high degree of suspicion. The family doctor continues to be one of the point people in the intervention process with drug abuse and dependence.

Psychiatric Emergencies

Emergency department physicians and new psychiatry residents soon realize that a large fraction of urgent and emergent medical care is purely psychiatric in nature. General medical practices and emergency departments are increasingly the most common venues for discussion of emotional issues. Although these problems may be approached in the same manner as other medical emergencies, there are some unique presentations and treatment challenges which can be summarized in four rules:

1. *Most cases that present as psychiatric emergencies are not.* It is not uncommon to find that an "acute depression" is only due to the latest in a long string of family arguments, or that an acute anxiety attack is the result of the patient's running out of benzodiazepines at 5:30 p.m. on a Friday afternoon. On the other hand, it is the apparent nonemergency that is the critical situation: A quiet young man reports to the emergency department with abdominal pain and has no abnormal findings. The nurse describes him as "confused" and closer examination reveals an acute paranoid psychosis with significant suicidal ideation.

2. *Psychiatric emergencies are almost always complicated.* They range from family conflicts to legal issues and medical complications. As

indicated in Rule 1, they are rarely what they seem and have a way of occurring when the schedule is full. The physician is required to be doctor, counselor, and sometimes prophet.

3. *Psychiatric emergencies always take time.* The patient in emotional distress or experiencing confusion needs time and attention. The more distressed the individual, the more convoluted the story. There may be more than one person to interview, including police, family, social workers, or clergy.

4. *Doctors cannot predict the future but will be asked to do so.* Often the question asked of the physician is, "What will this person be most likely to do over the next few hours?" You may be asked to evaluate suicidality or dangerousness. A family may want assurances about the course of a depression or a nurse may want to know what behavior to expect from an agitated postoperative patient. The prognosis for a medical condition may be an extremely difficult call, and predicting human behavior is even more complex, yet is routinely required in psychiatric situations.

Definitions

In the emergency department, decisions about diagnosis and treatment are frequently made simultaneously. In the acute psychiatric conditions it is helpful to have a decision process that is both practical and efficient, directed at the kinds of diagnoses that present urgently. Cases may be divided into three categories that share similar treatment approaches: cognitive or behavioral; interpersonal; and dysphoric disorders.

Cognitive and/or behavioral problems imply a disturbance in the patient's thinking or actions. These patients are usually brought to medical attention by someone else rather than by any significant insight on the part of the patient. The presenting problem may be bizarre behavior, violence, or confused or impaired thinking. Diagnoses include the schizophrenias, delirium, dementia, drug intoxication or withdrawal, neurologic disorders, metabolic dysfunction, and adverse drug reactions. A medical evaluation is necessary and behavior control is usually required. The primary medications are the phenothiazines, and in drug withdrawal, the benzodiazepines. Hospitalization is usually indicated, and in many cases a transfer to a psychiatric facility is necessary. Outside information may be critical in making the correct diagnosis. The advice of social service agencies should be sought to clarify issues of informed consent and voluntary versus involuntary care.

Interpersonal issues are perhaps the most common and encompass a broad range of problems. These include marital conflict; broken friendships and romances, which often lead to suicide attempts; depression secondary to a death or lost employment; job or home stress; and pressures of medical illness. These individuals may appear extremely distraught; they may defer the real reason for the visit until the last moment; and they routinely require the most time and the most listening. A suicide assessment is essential, and benzodiazepines are helpful. Inpatient care is a considered judgment, and a referral to a counselor may help determine whether the patient has the desire to get help or whether he is feeling hopeless and suicidal. Treatment primarily involves empathetic listening and referral to appropriate counselors or a return visit to your office, sometimes with a verbal contract with the patient to avoid self-harm or to call for help if needed.

Dysphoric disorders imply a subjective discomfort on the part of the patient. These individuals most often are self-referred and are in great emotional turmoil. As opposed to patients with interpersonal distress, they are more aware of their own symptoms than the causes. They may be suffering from major depressive disorders, anxiety states, panic attacks, obsessions, or psychosomatic symptoms. These are the anxiety disorders presenting as acute myocardial infarctions, the insomnias, the seriously suicidal patient, the anxious somaticizing patient, or the "burn out." They are motivated to obtain care but the diagnosis is not often obvious. Suicide risk is often high. The antidepressants are the most common medications; hospitalization is dependent on the severity of the symptoms. Close follow-up is important and the prognosis is quite good with treatment.

Evaluation of Suicide Risk

One of the most difficult tasks in the emergency setting is the assessment of suicide risk. The following points provide some guidance, but it is impossible to predict risk accurately in all situations.

- Take all suicide threats seriously. Even obvious gesturers make fatal mistakes.
- Listen, and ask questions about suicide ideation or previous attempts.
- Evaluate any plans for potential lethality and if possible contract with the patient to remove those items from the environment.
- Ask about any friends or relatives who may have committed suicide. Modeling behavior is very significant.
- Assess the support system. The more alone the patient is, the more likely a suicide attempt.
- Ask about alcohol use. Alcohol is a major factor in many suicides and alcoholics are at higher risk.
- Look for a major depressive disorder.
- Men are at higher risk for a successful suicide, though they attempt less often.
- Ask about recent losses of close friends and family. If you are seriously concerned about the risk, share this with the patient's family. Confidentiality is waived if there is a serious risk to life and limb.
- Do not be afraid to hospitalize even if a hold order is required. A hospital stay of only a few days may allow for further evaluation and may convince the patient that he or she has more of a support system than previously realized.

Finally, there are two dissimilar but important points to remember when confronting a psychiatric emergency. The first is that we, as physicians, often create such emergencies through the use of medications or because of a lack of sensitivity. A patient may come in panic stricken because of a diagnosis or treatment recommendation rendered in a cavalier fashion. The medications we prescribe may create anxiety, severe depression, or worrisome physical symptoms. It then becomes our responsibility to withdraw or change treatment. Discontinuing a medication can be as active a measure as starting one.

Secondly, it is a sad but true fact that emergency departments and all medical facilities are becoming more dangerous places to work, even in rural America. If you have any concerns about a patient or family member presenting a risk of violence, please take precautions. Consider having an emergency alert plan at your hospital or clinic, and remember that a reasonable degree of suspicion is your best defense.

Summary

Mental health care is virtually always a partnership in which the rural physician not only plays a role, but may in many cases be the first one on the scene. Considering that unique position and the sheer numbers of people that enter a medical office with either a primary or secondary psychiatric diagnosis, a knowledge of these disorders and their treatment is an absolute necessity. Beyond that necessity mental health is a rewarding area of practice where science, art, and compassion for people comfortably meet.

Recommended Reading

Buchsbaum, D. G., Buchanan, R. G., Centor, R. M., Schnoll, S. H., & Lawton, M. J. (1991). Screening for alcohol abuse using CAGE scores and likelihood ratios. *Annals of Internal Medicine, 115,* 774-777.

Greist, J. H. (1984). *Depression and its treatment: Help for the nation's #1 mental problem.* Washington, DC: American Psychiatric Press.

Hacket, T., & Cassem, N. (1987). *Massachusetts General Hospital handbook of general psychiatry.* Littleton, MA: PSG Publishing.

Hyman, S. E. (1984). *Manual of psychiatric emergencies.* Boston: Little, Brown.

Kline, N. S. (1974). *From Sad to glad: Kline on depression.* New York: Putnam.

Mace, N. L. (1981). *The thirty-six hour day: A family guide to caring for persons with Alzheimer's disease, related dementing illnesses, and memory loss later in life.* Baltimore, MD: Johns Hopkins University Press.

Mayfield, D., McLeod, G., & Hall, P. (1974). The CAGE questionnaire: Validation of a new alcoholism screening instrument. *American Journal of Psychiatry, 131,* 1121-1123.

Torrey, E. F. (1988). *Surviving schizophrenia: A famil16y manual.* New York: Perennial Library.

Patient Education Materials

Dean Foundation
8000 Excelsior Drive, Suite 203
Madison, WI 53717
(Anxiety disorders, bipolar disorders, and medication information)

American Psychiatric Press
1400 K Street NW
Washington, DC 20005
(Texts, patient pamphlets, DSM-III-R materials)

9
■ ■ ■

Environmental Hazards

BARBARA P. YAWN

Introduction

Many hazards and rewards of rural life come from the lack of "civilization": rugged country, great distances between health care facilities, and poorly maintained roads. But some of the hazards of rural life also come from "civilization." These hazards include environmental toxins. This chapter will present information on four environmental toxins. Although these are only a representative sample, the reference list provides resources to find out about others. Acute poisonings from materials such as herbicides and chemical products will not be covered. Information on those problems is usually readily available from the package or can be obtained quickly from "hot lines" maintained by the manufacturers. The toxins presented here are toxins that become part of our environment and may be difficult to identify if they are not included in your differential diagnosis.

Nitrates and Nitrites

Case Report

A 6-week-old infant is brought for well-child care. The pregnancy was uncomplicated and the child was delivered at term. She is bottle fed. The mother's only concern is an occasional blue color of the lips and ears. The exam shows the child to be gaining weight a little slowly but no physical abnormalities can be found. You encourage the parents to increase feedings.

The parents return for an emergency appointment 3 weeks later. The child is crying constantly, she has a tachycardia (140 beats per minute), and is lethargic and cyanotic. The central cyanosis does not improve with 100% oxygen for 1 hour.

This child does not have cardiac disease; she has methemoglobinemia from nitrate exposure. The clue is the bottle feeding and the lack of improvement of the central cyanosis with 100% oxygen in a child with no previous signs of heart disease.

Source of the Toxin

Nitrates are naturally occurring inorganic compounds that are part of the nitrogen cycle. They are likely to contaminate shallow, rural domestic wells, especially in areas where nitrogen-based fertilizers are in widespread use. Seepage from septic tank systems can exacerbate the problem. Nitrites can be found in foodstuffs, especially homemade deer sausage preserved with nitrites. Deliberate abuse of amyl, butyl, or isobutyl nitrites (known as snappers, poppers, or rushes) can also result in acute poisoning. A rare cause of toxicity is topical silver nitrate used in burn therapy over large areas in young children.

Who Is at Risk?

Infants less than 4 months old are at the highest risk. They have a higher gut pH and more fetal hemoglobin. Both result in greater toxicity and more methemoglobinemia. About 1% to 2% of all infants are exposed to drinking water with high levels of nitrates. The exposure rate is higher in rural areas.

Effects of the Toxin

The conversion of hemoglobin to methemoglobin is the major form of toxicity. Methemoglobin does not easily release its oxygen to the tissue and cyanosis and oxygen deprivation are the results. An occasional case of hemolytic anemia can also be seen.

- Cyanosis begins at methemoglobin levels of 10% to 20%.
- Central nervous system depression and dyspnea are usually seen next at levels of 20% to 45%.
- Hypotension, shock, cardiac arrhythmias, and coma may result in the most severe cases (45%-55% methemoglobinemia).
- Death is likely at levels above 70%.

Diagnosis

There are no useful direct measurements of nitrate in blood or urine. Blood methemoglobin levels must be measured. Measurement of oxygen saturation can be important clinically but is nonspecific.

Treatment

For very mild cases oxygen therapy and removal of the exposure may be sufficient. Methylene blue is an effective antidote when given intravenously. The Centers for Disease Control and Prevention (CDC) recommends 0.1 to 0.2 milliliters per kilogram of body weight in a 1% saline solution given intravenously over 5 to 10 minutes. Methylene blue should not be given to people with glucose-6-phosphate dehydrogenase deficiency. The cyanosis usually improves within 5 to 10 minutes. Further therapy can be done following consultation with the CDC or a toxicologist. Acute treatment alone is insufficient. The exposure source must be found and removed.

Lead Toxicity

Case Report

The Hones family has three children between the ages of 1 and 6 years of age. The 6-year-old is having trouble in school that has been diagnosed as a learning disability. The other children are also showing signs of developmental delay. This seems strange to the parents, who are both college educated and know of no family history of learning disabilities. The school has done extensive educational testing and suggests that all the children have medical evaluations. You do the evaluations and find that all three children indeed have developmental delays and mild anemia. Blood tests return 2 weeks later and are abnormal.

These children have lead toxicity. The parents also have elevated serum lead levels. They live in a farm house listed on the national register of historic homes. They have spent the past 8 years refurbishing the large three-story house and the barn. The children's bedrooms required scraping many coats of paint.

The children's lead levels are all in the range of 35 to 45 micrograms per deciliter. It is likely that the children were first exposed in utero and have been continuously reexposed through the dust and air contamination associated with the remodeling.

Definition of the Problem

Lead toxicity is the most common chronic disease of children, affecting as many as 17% of all children. Rural children are the least likely to be affected but still have rates of elevated lead levels as high in 46% in the poorest blacks, 19% in the poorest whites, and 5% in the white children of middle-class families. As recently as 1970, lead toxicity was defined by blood levels greater than 60 mcg/dl; these levels are associated with clinically apparent signs and symptoms such as vomiting, abdominal pain, irritability, and overt behavioral changes. Levels in this range could result in seizures, coma, or even death. Before 1975, subtle but serious and permanent neuropsychologic sequelae were thought to occur at lead levels above 40 mcg/dl. In 1975, maximum recommended levels were lowered to 30 mcg/dl, and in 1985 to 25 mcg/dl. Additional studies completed since 1985 suggest that levels of 10 to 15 mcg/dl can result in impaired cognitive and behavioral development. The newest CDC guidelines released in 1991 lowered the level for intervention to 10 mcg/dl of lead.

Source of the Toxin

The most common source of lead is paint made before 1977. Lead paint is in 52% of housing units in the United States. Lead-based paint is the most common source of lead in children with lead poisoning and it also contributes significantly to other sources of lead such as lead contaminated household dust and soil. Although paint in low-income housing is the most likely source of lead, many nonpoor children are exposed to dangerous quantities of lead during the remodeling and rehabilitation of older homes. Lead in dust and soil is a big problem for toddlers who are likely to play in the dirt. Airborne lead comes from stationary sources such as smelters and refineries and from mobile sources such as leaded gasoline. Even with removal of lead from paint and gasoline, lead remains in the soil and on walls of houses and old buildings.

Who Is at Risk?

Children from before birth to age 6 are at greatest risk of lead toxicity. Lead freely crosses the placenta and accumulates in the developing fetus. Many infants are born with significant lead burdens. After birth most lead enters the system through the gastrointestinal tract. Iron deficiency anemia increases the rate of absorption of lead from the GI tract. Lead in the body is distributed among three compartments of the body: the blood, the central nervous system, and the skeletal system. The levels in the three systems equilibrate.

Effects of the Toxin

Exposure to high lead levels can result in acute encephalopathy and persistent problems such as mental retardation, seizures, and behavioral dysfunction. Lead is a neurotoxin. Earlier exposure results in more severe defects and children in more disadvantaged environments are more likely to be affected. Even low levels of 10 to 15 mcg/dl can lead to reduced reaction times, lower ratings on classroom behavior, and a reduced intelligence quotient.

Diagnosis

Lead toxicity is diagnosed by measuring serum lead levels. Erythrocyte protoporphyrin (EP) is inadequate for screening as are other older tests such as basophilic stippling of red cells. Any serum lead level greater than 10 mcg/dl should be considered abnormal. An elevated serum lead level can be seen with acute toxicity. For children with levels above 25 to 30 mcg/dl, a combination of the elevated serum lead level and abnormal EP suggests chronic lead toxicity. Calcium disodium versenate (EDTA) provocative testing can also be useful. EDTA increases the leaching of lead from the skeletal system and will increase urine excretion of lead. The mobilization test reflects the overall body lead burden. This test is particularly helpful for patients with levels of 25 to 45 mcg/dl in which full chelation therapy may be useful.

The CDC currently recommends risk assessment in all children age 6 months and above. Assessment includes the following questions:

- Does the child live or regularly visit a house with peeling or chipping paint built before 1960? This includes day-care centers, preschool areas, and baby-sitter's home.
- Does the child live in or visit a house built before 1960 where renovation has been done, is being done, or is being planned?
- Does the child live with anyone with a lead level above 15 mcg/dl?

A positive answer to any of these questions requires a serum lead level. Any elevated capillary lead level must be confirmed by venous blood because skin or surface contamination may falsely elevate the level.

Treatment

Any child with lead levels above 10 to 15 mcg/dl must have identification of the environmental sources leading to the lead poisoning. The most important intervention at this level is modification of the environment to eliminate ongoing exposure and absorption of lead. Lead paint may not need to be removed because removal may exacerbate the existing lead hazard. Lead abatement should be done by professionals approved for lead control. Dust control can be done with frequent dusting with a damp cloth. Children must be removed from the environment when lead is being removed.

Dietary therapy includes a diet rich in iron, calcium, and zinc for children with levels above 15 mcg/dl. In children with even a minimally elevated lead level, iron deficiency should be identified and treated because a deficiency of iron increases the absorption of lead from the GI tract.

Dimercaptopropanol (BAL) is used for acute lead poisoning. Chelation therapy with EDTA is used in the treatment of children with chronic lead toxicity and levels greater than 45 mcg/dl. Chelation therapy in children with levels lower than 45 mcg/dl is controversial. Oral D-penicillamine has been used in children with levels from 20 to 40 mcg/dl but has many side effects; 2,3-Dimercaptosuccinic acid (DMSA) is an oral chelating agent that appears to be as effective as penicillamine and has fewer side effects. No studies have shown benefit from intravenous or oral chelation therapy for children with lead levels less than 25 mcg/dl.

Chronic Arsenic Toxicity

Case Report

A 60-year-old carpenter comes to your office for evaluation of numbness and tingling in his toes and fingertips. The symptoms have progressed slowly over the past few weeks and now include a burning and painful sensation in addition to the tingling. He has no ataxia, gastrointestinal, genitourinary, or visual symptoms. Although he did have a flu-like episode 4 months ago, he currently has no headaches, back or neck pain, or confusion.

The carpenter lives in a log cabin he built 10 years ago, next to the site of the tiny cabin he had built for himself 30 years earlier. He has a wood burning stove and prides himself on his wilderness lifestyle. He does not drink alcohol or smoke and takes no medications.

Examination reveals decreased sensation and proprioception over the hands and feet. Reflexes are absent at the ankles and 1+ at the knees and elbows. He has brown patches of hyperpigmentation and the palms and soles of his feet show hyperkeratotic lesions. He has a macrocytic anemia, increased eosinophils, and mildly elevated liver function tests.

Like most cases of chronic arsenic poisoning this is not an easy diagnosis. The source of the arsenic is usually difficult to discover and in this case is the burning of preserved wood used to build the first cabin and now used in the fireplace.

Source of the Toxin

Environmental sources of arsenic exposure are food, particularly fish, kelp, and wines; medicinals including naturopathic remedies and folk remedies; commercial products like wood preservatives, pesticides, herbicides, fungicides, and cattle and sheep dips; and industrial processes such as burning fossil fuels. Since 1987, 74% of the arsenic used in the United States is used in wood preservatives. Well water may be contaminated in some rural areas of the northwest and southwest United States and Alaska.

Who Is at Risk?

Industrial exposure from burning coal, use of preserved wood in a home fireplace, drinking contaminated ground water, and eating large amounts of contaminated seafood put many rural and wilderness residents at risk. Arsenic also crosses the placenta, and the fetus may be affected.

Effects of the Toxin

Because arsenic inhibits enzymes it affects almost all organ systems. Chronic arsenic toxicity is associated with lung and skin cancers, chronic renal failure, and peripheral vascular changes such as Raynaud's phenomenon. Acute arsenic toxicity is associated with hepatic damage, renal failure, diffuse capillary leakage, cardiomyopathy, peripheral neuropathy, and skin changes. Plantar hyperkeratosis that may progress to malignancy and patchy hyperpigmentation are the most common skin changes. Latency for skin and lung cancer may be decades.

Diagnosis

Acute exposure can be identified by urine arsenic levels. Chronic exposure is usually diagnosed by the typical patterns of symptoms and urine arsenic levels or arsenic levels in hair and nails. Hair and nail arsenic levels must be interpreted with care because they can be affected by direct contamination from smoke containing arsenic. Identifying the source and suspecting arsenic as the culprit may be the most difficult parts of the diagnostic process.

Treatment

Acute exposure is best treated with gut decontamination and stabilization of the patient. Administration of the chelating agent 2,3-dimercaptopropanol can be helpful within the first few hours of exposure. Consultation with a regional poison control center will be important in determining dosage and timing. Chronic exposure is best treated with supportive measures and removal of the source. Chelating agents are not helpful in treating established neuropathy. Improvement may take months and the patient may never return to baseline functioning.

Asbestos

Case Report

A 12-year-old boy is brought to your office complaining of trouble playing basketball. He is unable to run due to shortness of breath. The mother says he has been complaining ever since school started and has had an occasional cough. He has no other symptoms such as fever or chest pain and no history of asthma or previous similar symptoms. He does have "hay fever" in the spring. The mother is concerned because the school has sent home letters saying that asbestos is being removed from the school's boiler room and gymnasium. The boy has been playing basketball in the gym.

Exam reveals no respiratory distress, no tachypnea, but expiratory wheezes throughout the lungs. Chest X ray is normal; forced expiratory volume in 1 second is 88% of the normal predicted value and forced vital capacity is 95% of predicted value.

Parents are concerned about asbestos in schools, but they should also investigate asbestos sources in homes and farm buildings. Many of these buildings are old and have crumbling insulation and cement. It is unlikely that this child has pulmonary disease related to exposure to asbestos in the school gym or at home. However, it is reasonable to recommend inspection of the home and farm site. Treatment for exercise-induced asthma would be appropriate while the investigation is carried out.

Exposure

Asbestos exposure is primarily through inhalation of airborne fibrous particles. Asbestos was used in almost all insulating materials made before 1975. Asbestos is not biodegradable because it does not burn, dissolve, or react with most chemicals. In commercial buildings it may be found in cement pipes, conduits for electrical wire, heat protective pads, roofing materials, and sealants. In homes it is used for furnace insulation, pipe or boiler insulation, sheet vinyl or floor tiles, shingles, textured acoustical ceiling tiles, and under sheet flooring. Air can become contaminated from damaged or crumbling materials in the home or work buildings. Removal of asbestos that is not damaged or crumbling may be more harmful than leaving it in place and watching it carefully for signs of deterioration.

Who Is at Risk?

Workers in the construction trade and the asbestos removal business are at the greatest risk. Workers can expose their families by bringing dust-covered clothes home. Cigarette smoking potentiates the adverse effects of asbestos exposure.

Effects of the Toxin

Asbestos exposure is cumulative because most of the inhaled particles remain in the lungs. The primary effects of asbestos are on the lung: asbestosis, mesothelioma, and lung cancer. *Asbestosis* is interstitial fibrosis of the pulmonary parenchyma. Latency from exposure to clinical presentation is usually 20 to 40 years with X-ray changes after 20 years. *Mesotheliomas* are diagnostic of asbestos exposure until proven otherwise. Pleural plaques may develop in chronic asbestos exposure and are not considered premalignant but are indicators of asbestos exposure. Latency for mesotheliomas and lung cancer is 10 to 30 years. Gastrointestinal and immune system effects have been noted.

Diagnosis

Asbestosis is diagnosed by X ray and lung findings of dry rales and progressive dyspnea in an exposed individual. Both the X ray and pulmonary function tests are important in diagnosis. The malignant lesions are best diagnosed by imaging procedures and direct biopsy. Because interstitial fibrosis and malignancy are unlikely to be curable, early suspicion and removal of the exposure are critical.

Treatment

Asbestosis is treated by aggressive management of pulmonary infections and avoidance of irritants such as cigarette smoke. Pleural plaques require no treatment except for observation for other effects of asbestos exposure. The cancers associated with asbestosis are aggressive and difficult to treat. Education and prevention are the best forms of therapy.

Summary

Environmental medicine is of increasing concern in our country. Air pollution is generally associated with urban centers. However, ground water pollution from farm chemicals, air and water pollution from deteriorating buildings, and air pollution from open burning of preserved woods and building materials is of increasing concern in rural and wilderness areas. Many of the pollutants are concentrated as they move up the food chain. Warnings on fish consumption from the Great Lakes, certain regions of the oceans, and even local small lakes and streams are evidence of this growing problem. In this chapter, four examples of toxins important to rural practitioners have been outlined. The reading list and resources give the address of the Agency for Toxic Substance and Disease Registry, which has a complete set of monographs on this subject. The monographs are well written and easy to read. Each includes a case report and continuing medical education credit is available.

Recommended Reading

Agocs, M. A., & Clarkson, T. (1990). *Case studies in environmental medicine: Mercury toxicity.* Atlanta, GA: U.S. Department of Health and Human Services, Public Health Services, Agency for Toxic Substances and Disease Registry.
Centers for Disease Control. (1991). *Preventing lead poisoning in young children: A statement by the Centers for Disease Control.* Atlanta, GA: U.S. Department of Health and Human Services, Public Health Service.

Demers, R., & Selikoff, I. (1990). *Case studies in environmental medicine: Asbestos toxicity.* Atlanta, GA: U.S. Department of Health and Human Services, Public Health Services, Agency for Toxic Substances and Disease Registry.

Kosnett, M. C., & Kreiss, K. (1990). *Case studies in environmental medicine: Arsenic toxicity.* Atlanta, GA: U.S. Department of Health and Human Services, Public Health Services, Agency for Toxic Substances and Disease Registry.

Needleman, H. L., & Gatsonis, C. A. (1990). Low-level lead exposure and the IQ of children: A meta-analysis of modern studies. *Journal of the American Medical Association, 263,* 673-678.

Needleman, H. L., Schell, A., Bellinger, D., Leviton, A., & Alfred, E. N. (1990). The long-term effects of exposure to low dose lead in childhood. *New England Journal of Medicine, 322,* 83-88.

Ziegler, E. E., Edwards, B. B., Jensen, R. L., Mahaffey, K. R., & Fomon, S. J. (1978). Absorption and retention of lead by infants. *Pediatric Research, 12,* 29-34.

Other Resources

Other case studies are available from:

Department of Health and Human Services
Public Health Service
Centers for Disease Control
Agency for Toxic Substances and Disease Registry
Atlanta, GA 30333

Topics include:

Polychlorinated Biphenyl (PCB) toxicity
Cadmium toxicity
Chromium toxicity
Cyanide toxicity
Vinyl Chloride toxicity
Methylene Chloride toxicity
Polynuclear Aromatic Hydrocarbon (PAH) toxicity
Trichloroethylene toxicity

Each booklet includes case reports and a posttest for continuing medical education credits.

10
■ ■ ■

Managing Trauma in the Rural Emergency Department:
Basic Organization

DAVID M. LARSON

Introduction

Caring for the critically injured patient in the community hospital emergency department can be very challenging. In the urban setting these patients are taken directly to a trauma center. However, in rural areas they present first to the community hospital where they must receive life-saving emergency and stabilization care before they can be transferred to an urban trauma center. Rural physicians may not opt out of emergency trauma care.

In this chapter we will discuss the general approach to the injured patient. With some adaptations, this approach can be used for all trauma patients, from patients with relatively minor injuries to those with severe life-threatening trauma. The emphasis will be on the management in the first hour ("The Golden Hour").

Rural emergency care involves much more than care rendered by the physician in the emergency department. The rural physician must provide leadership in developing an organized, systematic approach to care for the injured that involves many other health care providers such as first responders, emergency medical technicians, and nurses. This chapter will also discuss the components of the rural Emergency Medical Services System and emphasize development of protocols for rural emergency departments.

Epidemiology of Rural Trauma

Trauma is the leading cause of death in persons under 38 years of age and the fourth leading cause of death in the United States. Motor vehicle crashes are by far the leading cause of accidental deaths. Even though 70% of all crashes occur in urban areas, 70% of all motor vehicle-related fatalities occur in the rural setting. Agriculture is currently rated as America's most dangerous industry. More than 1,000 farmers are killed each year in the United States. In 1991, the state of Iowa reported 68 fatalities and 2,599 injuries from farm-related accidents (Smith, 1987).

Trauma deaths occur in a trimodal distribution. The first peak (50%) includes deaths that occur in the first few minutes, often due to unsalvageable injuries such as heart and great vessel lacerations, decapitations, and severe brain or high spinal cord injuries. The second peak of deaths (30%) falls within minutes to a few hours after the accident. Deaths during this period are often due to hypovolemia and respiratory failure. This time period is often referred to as the "Golden Hour" because it is a period of time in which definitive emergency care must be provided or death will ensue. The third peak of deaths (20%) occurs several days to weeks after the injury, possibly due to multi-organ failure or sepsis (Trunkey, 1983).

The types of injuries seen in the rural hospital emergency departments are somewhat different than those in the urban centers. Although most serious injuries are due to blunt trauma resulting from motor vehicle crashes, significant trauma also results from falls, assaults, farm animal- and machinery-related injuries, recreational vehicle injuries (boats, all-terrain vehicles, snowmobiles), and gunshot wounds from hunting accidents. The rural practitioner is faced with the same severity of injuries that present to the urban trauma center but with decreased frequency.

Unique Problems of Rural Trauma

The chances of dying from a given injury are greater in the rural setting compared to the urban setting. There are a number of reasons for this, including:

- isolation resulting in extended periods of time before discovery of the injury
- greater distances between the scene and the hospital
- prehospital care provided by volunteers with only basic emergency medical skills
- emergency departments staffed by primary care physicians who may not have the surgical skills needed for managing critically injured trauma patients
- delays in treatment if physicians and ancillary staff are not "in-house"
- small numbers of critically injured accident victims, making it difficult to maintain skills

Strategies can be developed to overcome some of these problems so that a rural medical community can deliver optimal care to the injured patient.

Understanding the Rural Trauma System

In each rural community, a designated physician must provide medical direction and leadership for the local trauma or emergency medical system (EMS) to assure that all components of the system are functioning and interrelating well. The components of the trauma system include:

- communications and dispatch
- first responder groups
- ambulance services
- trauma facilities

Communications and Dispatch: Access to Emergency Care

Public Safety Answering Point (PSAP) dispatchers should be easily accessed through the 911 system. Dispatchers must know the resources and facilities for their region. The emergency medical dispatcher is a key player in the emergency medical system (Clawson, 1981).

First Responder Groups. A first responder is an individual who has successfully completed the 40-hour Department of Transportation First Responder Course or its equivalent and is a member of an organized group that is dispatched to the scene of an injury or illness in the prehospital setting. Most first responder groups are affiliated with a fire department, law enforcement agency, or a licensed ambulance service. Especially in rural areas, where ambulances may be responding from a nearby city, first responder units play an essential role by providing initial stabilization procedures. First responders perform cardiopulmonary resuscitation, hemorrhage control, splinting, and in some cases automatic defibrillation.

Ambulance Services. There are several levels of prehospital care providers that staff ambulance services. The Department of Transportation (DOT) has published three sets of curricula for emergency medical technicians (EMT): the EMT-Basic (or EMT-A), the EMT-Intermediate (EMT-I), and the EMT-Paramedic (EMT-P). The EMT-Basic curriculum usually involves 100-115 hours of training. These skills include patient assessments, administration of oxygen, positive pressure ventilation, automatic defibrillation, pneumatic antishock garment (PASG) application, and spinal immobilization. The EMT-I curriculum requires a variable number of additional hours of training and may allow intravenous line placement, limited drug use, and advanced airway management. The EMT-P course provides 700-1,000 hours of training. Additional skills include endotracheal intubation, cardiac monitoring, defibrillation, cardioversion, cardiac drug use, needle thoracostomy, and needle cricothyrotomy.

Most rural ambulance services are basic life-support services and are staffed by EMTs (basic or intermediate), and many times the personnel are volunteers. In general, $200,000 to $300,000 per year is required to run a 24-hour advanced life-support vehicle. Because of the low volume of activity in many rural areas such a service becomes impractical.

Trauma Facilities. The Committee on Trauma of the American College of Surgeons (1990) has defined levels of trauma facilities. The Level I facility is a tertiary hospital capable of providing total care for the most critically injured. A Level II trauma hospital serves as a community trauma center. This facility has the capability of handling most trauma cases. The Level III facility is a rural trauma hospital that has made a maximum commitment to trauma care commensurate with its local resources. This facility must have transfer agreements and protocols as it may not have many of the resources associated with a Level I or II hospital.

Preparations Before the Accident

One of the most important elements in managing a critically injured patient is avoiding delays in getting the patient to definitive care. Preparation and organization of the emergency department and staff are the keys to providing prompt care (Campbell, 1988).

Preparing the Resuscitation Area

The resuscitation area should be a room that can be easily accessed from the ambulance entrance but set apart from the flow of other patients and visitors. In small hospitals with a single emergency room, some arrangements must be made to close off and secure that room when caring for a critically injured patient. A nearby family room with comfortable furnishings should be available, attended by a social worker or chaplain.

Table 10.1 lists the equipment and drugs that should be available. These should be catalogued and stored in an easily accessible location.

Preparing the Staff

The best way to prepare the emergency medical staff is through education. The 16-hour Advanced Trauma Life Support (ATLS) Course sponsored by the American College of Surgeons was especially designed for the rural practitioner. Information regarding the ATLS Course may be obtained by contacting the American College of Surgeons or one of the Regional Trauma Centers. The Trauma Nurse Core Curriculum sponsored by the Emergency Nurse Association is an equivalent course for nurses. The Basic Trauma Life Support Course sponsored by the American College of Emergency Physicians is intended for EMTs.

Table 10.1 Required Emergency Department Equipment and Drugs

Airway Cart
  oropharyngeal/nasopharyngeal airways, endotracheal tubes, laryngo-
  scope, suction catheters, stylets, tracheostomy tubes, tape, benzoin, jaw
  spreader, McGill forceps, lidocaine spray
Cricothyrotomy Tray
  scalpel blade and handle, tracheal hook, Trousseau dilator, #4 Shiley
  tracheostomy tubes
Oxygen: 2 Outlets
  adapter for transtracheal needle ventilation
  Elder valve
Suction: 2-3 Vacuum Outlets
  Yankauer or dental tip suction catheter
  tracheal suction
  chest tube or nasogastric suction
Cardiac monitor/defibrillator/external pacemaker
Automatic blood pressure monitor
Pulse oximeter
End tidal CO_2 monitor
Intravenous catheters and crystalloid
High-volume trauma IV tubing
6-8 French high-volume infusion catheters
Central venous pressure catheter trays
Blood and fluid warmer
PASG (MAST) trousers
IV pumps
Interosseous infusion needles
Chest tube trays
Thoracotomy tray
Peritoneal lavage catheters
Heat lamps
Hypothermia thermometer
Humidified oxygen warming device
Nasogastric tubes
Foley catheters
Fax machine
Drugs
  Mannitol
  SoluMedrol
  Succinylcholine
  Vercuronium or pancuronium
  Sodium pentothal
  Haloperidol or droperidol
  Midazolam, diazepam
  Morphine sulfate, fentanyl
  Lidocaine
Parenteral antibiotics
Tetanus Immune Globulin, tetanus toxoid
Pediatric drug dosing charts
Portable X-ray machine and lead-lined aprons

Multidisciplinary case conferences where trauma cases are presented and discussed allow providers to learn from the experiences of their colleagues. Periodic mock trauma codes similar to the "Moulage Scenarios" from the ATLS course may also be useful.

The Trauma Protocol

As soon as a critically injured trauma patient is encountered by the First Responders or EMTs, the trauma system must be alerted. This involves activation of the trauma team at the local hospital, alerting the regional trauma center, and perhaps initiating a response by the aeromedical transport team in preparation for inter-facility transfer. Only 10%-15% of trauma patients require the entire system, specifically those with respiratory difficulty, shock, and an altered level of consciousness.

The EMT should immediately notify the hospital and perform a rapid extrication and "load and go." The scene time should be less than 10 minutes if possible. Some local systems use a code word such as "Code Red" or "Trauma Code" in order to enhance communication between the hospital and the scene. These codes require the hospital to mobilize and assemble the trauma team.

The Rural Hospital Trauma Team

The **physician team leader** could be a general surgeon if available. If a surgeon is not available, a primary care or emergency physician who has had Advanced Trauma Life Support training should be selected.

A **second physician** should be available to assist with airway procedures, chest tube placement, or central venous line insertion.

Two registered nurses with critical care experience are needed: The first nurse maintains and records all intravenous fluids and medications given, while the second nurse obtains supplies and assists with procedures.

The **anesthetist** assists with airway management and IV placement.

The **radiology technician** obtains high-priority radiographs such as lateral cervical spine, chest, and pelvic films.

The **laboratory technician** draws a trauma battery that may include type and crossmatch, hemoglobin and hematocrit, urinalysis, glucose, arterial blood gases, and electrolytes.

The **social worker** offers support and communicates with family members.

The **recorder** may be an extra nurse or secretary who will record all pertinent clinical information on a trauma flow sheet.

The **trauma team** should be assembled in the resuscitation area before the patient's arrival. After radio communication with the EMTs at the scene, the team leader should be able to anticipate a management plan, assign a role to each team member, and consider transport to another facility.

Approach to the Injured Patient

It is essential that the physician have a systematic approach when evaluating and resuscitating a trauma patient (Campbell, 1988). The first question to ask obviously is: "What happened?" Understanding the kinetics of trauma will help the physician to anticipate certain types of injuries and to recognize a high likelihood of significant injuries that may require transfer to a regional trauma center. Types of trauma that result in a high probability of serious injury include:

- a fall from greater than 15 feet
- an automobile crash or pedestrian injury with a vehicle velocity of greater than 25 miles per hour
- rearward displacement of the front axle or front of the car by more than 20 inches
- ejection of the victim from the vehicle
- death of an occupant in the same car

A Polaroid picture of the scene can help the physician in the emergency department to assess the probability of severe injuries.

Primary care physicians are trained to take a complete history, perform a thorough physical examination, obtain appropriate laboratory and radiology studies, and then render treatment. The approach to the trauma patient is different. The assessment and the resuscitation phases of trauma care occur simultaneously. The team leader must promptly and accurately carry out a primary survey and delegate the appropriate treatment to the other members of the team (Table 10.2).

Table 10.2 Primary Survey of the Critically Injured Patient

1. Is the C-spine immobilized	Control C-spine
2. Is the patient awake? Ask "How are you?" and "What happened?"	If no: suction airway, place naso- pharyngeal or oropharyngeal airway; expose chest; cut off clothing
3. Is the airway open and clear?	Give oxygen by rebreather mask for shock, head injury, or respiratory difficulty
4. Are the respiratory rate and tidal volume adequate? Look, listen, and feel chest. Rate too fast (> 20)? Rate too slow (< 12)?	Assist ventilation with bag mask valve Attach ECG monitor Attach pulse oximeter
5. Does the patient need to be intubated? Now? Later?	Prepare for intubation
6. Is there evidence of shock? —palpate carotid and radial pulse, noting rate and strength —skin color —capillary refill	Start two large bore intravenous lines (14-16 ga) with warm crystalloid Type and cross match blood
7. Is the trachea midline?	If no, consider tension pneumothorax
8. Are the neck veins distended?	If yes, consider tension pneumothorax or pericardial tamponade
9. Any active bleeding?	Apply direct pressure to control bleeding
10. Does the patient need MAST suit applied?	Perform MAST survey, examine abdo- men, pelvis, and lower extremities
11. What is the patient's level of responsiveness? —alert —responds to verbal stimuli —responds to painful stimuli —unresponsive	
12. Decision to transfer to trauma center	Make arrangements for mode of transfer Contact trauma center
OR	
go to operating room at your hospital	operating room notified and staff available

After the primary survey is completed, the physician initiates a secondary survey (Table 10.3) to visualize and palpate the patient from head to toe. Simultaneously, other team members are delegated to perform other resuscitation and diagnostic procedures.

After the primary and secondary surveys are completed, the team should try to obtain further information about the patient's medical history by using the mnemonic "AMPLE":

A: Allergies
M: Medication
P: Past Illness
L: Last meal
E: Events/environment related to injury

Family and friends may be able to provide this vital information if the patient cannot respond.

In most circumstances, the evaluation and stabilization of the injured patient should not take longer than 45-60 minutes. There should be no delays due to performing procedures or X rays that will not immediately affect the patient's care.

Refer to Table 10.4 for interhospital transfer criteria. If transfer to another facility is indicated, use the following checklist to assure that the basic elements of care have been completed.

1. Secured airway to include endotracheal intubation when indicated. This includes head injury with a Glasgow Coma Scale of 10 or less, respiratory distress, and burns with potential for upper airway swelling.
2. External bleeding controlled.
3. Two large bore intravenous lines with crystalloid infusion.
4. Blood for replacement as needed.
5. Nasogastric tube to prevent aspiration.
6. Indwelling urinary catheter to monitor urine output.
7. Chest tube inserted for any trauma patient with pneumothorax or hemothorax.
8. Radiographs of lateral cervical spine, chest, and pelvis if time permits.
9. Secured cervical, thoracic, and lumbar spine.
10. Arterial blood gas determination, urinalysis, hemoglobin.
11. Splinting of fractures as appropriate.

Table 10.3 Secondary Survey of the Critically Injured Patient

Team Leader Examination and Findings	Response Delegate Procedures
HEAD	
Look: for battle signs, raccoon's eyes, blood from ears or nose, pupil size and reaction to light, cyanosis, pallor	Take BP, HR, RR, temp. Use automatic BP cuff
Palpate: for lacerations, tenderness, facial fractures	Arterial blood gases
Reassess: airway	
NECK	
Look: for bruising, penetrating injury	Lateral C-spine X ray
Palpate: for tenderness, crepitus, midline trachea	
Reassess: airway	
CHEST	
Look: for bruising, penetrations, paradoxical motions	Chest X ray
Palpate: for crepitus, tenderness, paradoxical motion	Insert chest tube for hemo-thorax or pneumothorax
Listen: for unequal breath sounds	
ABDOMEN	
Look: for bruising, distention, penetration	Insert NG tube
Palpate: for tenderness, rigidity	
RECTUM	
Note: sphincter tone	Insert Foley catheter
Palpate: for pelvic fracture, high riding prostate	
PELVIS	
Palpate: for instability, tenderness	AP pelvis X ray
EXTREMITIES	
Look: for deformities, bruising, penetration, lacerations	Splint fracture MAST suit for femur or pelvic fractures
Palpate: for tenderness, instability	CBC, electrolytes, UA
NEUROLOGIC	
Check pupils: response to light, equal?	Antibiotics, tetanus when indicated
Levels of responsiveness: —Glasgow Coma Scale	
Motor and sensory evaluation of extremities —look for lateralized weakness	

Table 10.4 Interhospital Transfer Criteria

CENTRAL NERVOUS SYSTEM
        Penetrating head injury or depressed skull fracture
        Open head injury with or without cerebrospinal fluid leak
        Glasgow Coma Scale < 13 or deterioration
        Lateralizing signs
        Spinal cord injury

CHEST
        Wide superior mediastinum
        Major chest wall injury
        Cardiac injury
        Patients who require protracted ventilation

PELVIS
        Unstable pelvic ring disruption
        Pelvic ring disruption with shock and evidence of continuing
            hemorrhage
        Open pelvic injury

MULTIPLE SYSTEM INJURY
        Severe face injury with head injury
        Chest injury with head injury
        Abdominal or pelvic injury with head injury
        Burns with associated injuries
        Multiple fractures

EVIDENCE OF HIGH-ENERGY IMPACT
        Auto crash or pedestrian injury with velocity > 25 miles per
            hour
        Rearward displacement of front axle or front of car (20 inches)
        Ejection of patient or rollover
        Death of occupant in same car

COMORBID FACTORS
        Age < 5 years or > 55 years
        Known cardiorespiratory or metabolic disease

SECONDARY DETERIORATION (LATE SEQUELAE)
        Mechanical ventilation required
        Sepsis
        Single or multiple organ system failure (deterioration in central
            nervous, cardiac, pulmonary, hepatic, renal, or coagulation
            systems)
        Major tissue necrosis

Summary

The basic structure of rural trauma management has been described, including organization of the emergency department and staff. The initial approach to the injured patient has been outlined, from the accident site to early stabilization of the patient in the emergency department. For hospitals with limited resources, basic requirements and criteria for transfer to a referral center were provided. The next chapter discusses specific problems in trauma management that the rural physician will encounter.

References

Campbell, J. E. (1988). *Basic trauma life support.* Englewood Cliffs, NJ: Prentice Hall.

Clawson, J. (1981). Dispatch priority training: Strengthening the weak link. *Journal of Emergency Medical Service, 6,* 32-36.

Committee on Trauma of the American College of Surgeons. (1990). *Resources for optimal care of the injured patient.* Chicago: American College of Surgeons.

Smith, N. (1987). The incidence of severe trauma in small rural hospitals. *Journal of Family Practice, 25,* 595-600.

Trunkey, D. D. (1983). Trauma. *Scientific American, 249,* 28-35.

Additional Reading

Caroline, N. (Ed.). (1987). *Emergency care in the streets.* Boston: Little, Brown.

Kuehl, A. (Ed.). (1989). *EMS medical directors handbook.* St. Louis: C. V. Mosby.

Other Resources

American College of Surgeons
55 E. Erie Street
Chicago, IL 60611
(Advanced Trauma Life Support Course)

American College of Emergency Physicians
P.O. Box 619911
Dallas, TX 75261
(Principles of EMS Systems)

Emergency Nurses Association
230 East Ohio
Suite 600
Chicago, IL 60611
(Trauma Nurse Core Curriculum)

11
■ ■ ■

Managing Trauma in the Rural Emergency Department:
Specific Problems

DAVID M. LARSON

Introduction

In the preceding chapter we discussed the basic organization of rural trauma services and emergency departments. The initial evaluation and management of the injured patient was also described. In this chapter we will outline in detail the management of four specific problems frequently encountered in acutely injured patients: airway management, shock, head injury, and amputation. We will also provide more details about the transfer procedure.

Airway Management

Airway management in the trauma patient can be the most difficult and the most important aspect of emergency trauma care (Walls, 1992). In cases where there is a significant head injury, absolute airway control via endotracheal intubation is essential. This may seem relatively easy in the flaccid, unresponsive patient; but it is very challenging in the hypotensive, combative, head-injured patient who may also have an unstable cervical spine injury.

During the primary survey, basic maneuvers are used to open and maintain the airway. This includes use of the chin lift or jaw thrust, taking care to maintain immobilization of the cervical spine. Blood, secretions, or emesis may need to be suctioned from the oropharynx using the tonsil tip or dental tip suction device. An oropharyngeal or nasopharyngeal airway may be inserted to keep the airway open in an obtunded patient. High flow oxygen should be administered using a nonrebreather mask or bag-valve device.

If it is noted in the primary survey that the patient is not ventilating adequately, ventilations must be assisted using a bag-valve-mask device. When giving positive pressure ventilations, air is forced into the oropharynx with pressures that inflate not only the trachea but the esophagus as well, leading to gastric insufflation. When this happens the patient develops gastric distension and is likely to vomit and is at risk for aspiration. This can be prevented by properly performing Sellick's maneuver when ventilating the patient.

Sellick's maneuver involves having an assistant place two fingers over the cricoid cartilage and apply pressure to displace it posteriorly. The cricoid cartilage, located about 1 centimeter below the thyroid cartilage (laryngeal prominence), is shaped like a signet ring with the ring anterior and the signet posterior. The esophagus lies directly posterior to the cricoid cartilage and is occluded by posterior displacement of the cricoid.

After performing these basic airway maneuvers during the primary survey the physician must next ask the question: "Does this patient need endotracheal intubation?" In the comatose patient with a Glasgow Coma Scale (GCS) score of 8 or less the answer is definitely "yes." The next question is: "Does the patient need to be intubated now or can we wait a few minutes in order to get a lateral cervical spine X ray?" In an apneic or hypoventilating trauma patient there may not be time to do a lateral cervical spine X ray. In this case the patient should be intubated using meticulous in-line cervical stabilization.

Deciding when or whether to intubate a poorly responsive but combative patient can be difficult. The patient might benefit from a neuroleptic drug such as haloperidol (0.1 mg/kg IV every 5-10 minutes up to a total dose of 0.5 mg/kg) or sedation with midazolam (0.01-0.1 mg/kg). This may allow better control of the patient and therefore allow time to x-ray the C-spine. If the patient is going to be transferred to another facility one may elect to intubate a patient with a GCS of 10 or less so that the airway is secure should the patient deteriorate en route. In cases where the decision may be difficult it would be worthwhile discussing it with the receiving trauma center.

There are three methods for performing endotracheal intubation: blind nasotracheal intubation, orotracheal intubation using rapid sequence induction (intubation), and cricothyrotomy. Percutaneous transtracheal jet ventilation may be used as a temporizing measure. Some other types of advanced airway techniques that have been described but will not be discussed here include fiber-optic guided intubation, use of a lighted stylet, digital intubation, and retrograde intubation over a catheter (Campbell, 1988).

Blind Nasotracheal Intubation

In the head injured patient, the disadvantages of this method probably outweigh the advantages. The proponents of this technique feel that there is better cervical spine control than with orotracheal intubation and have therefore recommended its use when there is an immediate need for an airway in the patient who is breathing and who may have cervical spine injury. This technique is relatively difficult. It may cause significant rises in intracranial pressure with stimulation of the upper airway and trachea. There is no good evidence that there is less mobility of the cervical spine than there is with orotracheal intubation using proper in-line manual cervical immobilization. For these reasons the author prefers orotracheal intubation using rapid sequence intubation.

Orotracheal Intubation With
Rapid Sequence Intubation

Rapid sequence induction (RSI) or "crash intubation" has traditionally been used by anesthesiologists in the operating room to intubate patients who have full stomachs and who are at risk for regurgitation and aspiration. This technique, which involves paralyzing and anesthetizing the patient simultaneously, has also been used successfully by physicians in the emergency department in trauma patients. The main advantage of RSI in the head-injured patient is that it prevents elevations in intracranial pressure caused by intubation. It also provides optimal conditions for intubations in extremely difficult patients such as those who may be combative or have clenched teeth.

Technique for RSI

1. Organize all equipment and medications.
2. Preoxygenate with 100% oxygen for 5 minutes if time permits; otherwise give 3-5 tidal volume breaths with bag-valve-mask.
3. Pretreat with lidocaine 1.0-1.5 mg/kg IV, 2 minutes prior to intubation. This prevents the rise in intracranial pressure with tracheal stimulation.
4. Pretreat with vercuronium or pancuronium 0.01 mg/kg IV, 2 minutes before intubation. This is a "defasciculating" dose that prevents fasciculations and the rise in intracranial pressure due to succinylcholine.
5. Paralyze with succinylcholine 1.5 mg/kg IV. The onset of paralysis is in 45-60 seconds and lasts 10 minutes. Pretreat with atropine 0.01 mg/kg IV in children; use this also in adults with the second or third dose of succinylcholine. Caution: This may cause hyperkalemia in patients with severe burns or soft tissue damage more than 24 hours old.
6. Induce anesthesia with sodium pentothal 3-5 mg/kg IV; onset of action is within 30 seconds. This reduces cerebral blood flow and therefore lowers intracranial pressure. It also lowers metabolic oxygen consumption. Caution: This drug acts as a myocardial depressant, so reduce the dose to 1.5-3 mg/kg in patients with borderline hemodynamic compromise. Do not use in hypotensive patients; consider another induction agent such as fentanyl 1.5-3 micrograms/kg IV.
7. Apply Sellick's maneuver as soon as the pentothal is given because the esophageal sphincter will be relaxed and the reflexes will be diminished. Continue until intubation is complete and the balloon is inflated.
8. Intubate 45-60 seconds after giving succinylcholine. DO NOT BAG THE PATIENT WHILE WAITING TO INTUBATE. If the patient was preoxygenated, you have several minutes to intubate.
9. After intubation, secure the tracheal tube. Obtain a chest X ray to confirm the tube position. Hyperventilate.
10. Give a longer acting paralytic agent (vercuronium 0.8-0.1 mg/kg IV, duration of action 25-30 minutes, or pancuronium 0.8-0.1 mg/kg IV, duration of action 60 minutes) as needed to transfer the patient.

Cricothyrotomy

The indication for this technique is the inability to intubate with other methods. Fracture of the larynx, massive facial trauma with severe swelling and bleeding obviating adequate visualization of the cords, or failure of attempted intubation are reasons for cricothyrotomy. This procedure is not recommended in children under 12 years old.

Properly defining the anatomy and locating the crycothyroid membrane are the keys to successful cricothyrotomy. The crycothyroid membrane is approximately 1 centimeter below the thyroid notch between the thyroid cartilage and the cricoid cartilage. It measures approximately 0.5 cm vertically by 1.5-2.0 cm horizontally.

Procedure for Cricothyrotomy

1. With the patient in the supine position, the neck is stabilized by an assistant. The neck is quickly prepped and draped.
2. Using the nondominant hand, the thyroid notch is identified and the thyroid cartilage is held firmly between the thumb and middle finger. The cricothyroid membrane is then palpated just caudal with the index finger of the nondominant hand.
3. With a # 11 blade, a 2-3 cm vertical midline incision is made over the cricothyroid membrane and carried down to the membrane.
4. The tracheal hook is inserted into the membrane with the operator's dominant hand and held securely in place with the other hand.
5. With a #11 blade, a stab incision is made horizontally through the cricothyroid membrane.
6. While continuing to hold the membrane steady with the tracheal hook, dilate the vertical dimension of the cricothyrotomy incision with the Trousseau dilator (or curved hemostat).
7. Insert a #4 Shiley tracheostomy tube (average adult size) into the opening through the cricothyroid membrane and direct it into the trachea caudally. After the tube has been inserted, remove the trocar and insert the inner cannula.
8. Inflate the cuff and ventilate the patient. If there is any question regarding proper placement into the trachea, pass a tracheal suction catheter through the tube; this should pass easily.
9. Obtain a chest X ray and secure the tube.

Shock

Shock is an abnormality of the circulatory system resulting in inadequate tissue perfusion. One of the mistakes that occasionally occurs in trauma care is the failure to recognize and adequately treat hypovolemic shock. The problem is not the failure to recognize shock in the hypotensive trauma patient, but rather the failure to recognize the signs of inadequate tissue perfusion in early shock. The trauma victim may lose up to 30% of his blood volume before a drop in systolic blood pressure occurs. The recognition and initial treatment of shock in the injured patient are vital to a successful outcome (Committee on Trauma of the American College of Surgeons [1988] provides a wealth of information).

Shock can be classified into four basic types: hypovolemic, cardiogenic, neurogenic, and septic. By far the most common type seen in the injured patient is hypovolemic shock due to hemorrhage. Cardiogenic shock may result from myocardial contusion, cardiac tamponade, myocardial infarction, or tension pneumothorax. Neurogenic shock results from spinal cord injuries, with loss of sympathetic tone, which is manifested by hypotension without compensatory tachycardia. Septic shock is rarely seen immediately after an injury.

Recognition of Shock

It is important to recognize the early clinical signs of shock. Hypovolemic shock secondary to hemorrhage will be used to exemplify the stages of shock:

- Class I Hemorrhage (early or mild): Up to 15% volume loss. There is a minimal increase in heart rate and no change in respiratory rate, pulse pressure, capillary refill, or blood pressure.
- Class II Hemorrhage (moderate): From 15% to 30% volume loss. Tachycardia, followed by a decrease in pulse pressure (systolic BP minus diastolic BP). Capillary refill is greater than 2 seconds. Respiratory rate begins to rise. Signs of anxiety may also be present. There is little or no change in urine output. There is still no drop in systolic blood pressure.
- Class III Hemorrhage (severe): From 30% to 40% volume loss. Systolic blood pressure now falls. In addition there is a marked tachycardia, tachypnea, and delayed capillary refill. Mental status changes

are present beginning with anxiety followed by confusion and eventually lethargy. Urine output also begins to drop.

- Class IV Hemorrhage (life threatening): Greater than 40% volume loss. Marked drop in blood pressure, tachycardia, tachypnea, and lethargy. A late, ominous sign is a decline in the heart rate reflecting a profound acidosis. This is a prearrest state.

The clinical signs of shock progress along a continuum depending on the degree of blood loss as well as the underlying physiologic status of the individual. For example, a 25% volume blood loss in a healthy 10-year-old will demonstrate a very different clinical picture than the same volume loss in a 70-year-old on beta-blockers.

The first priority in managing shock is an adequate airway and ventilation including high-flow oxygen (100%). Vascular access should be accomplished with two large-bore catheters (at least 16 gauge). Peripheral antecubital veins are preferred over central venous access for volume replacement. In cases of severe hemorrhage, peripheral intravenous catheters can be converted to high-volume infusion catheters using the Seldinger technique. In life-threatening hemorrhage, high-volume introducer catheters may be inserted into central veins such as subclavian, internal jugular, or femoral veins. Special high-volume intravenous tubing is also available.

When giving large amounts of blood or fluid replacement it is best to warm the fluids first in order to prevent iatrogenic hypothermia. A fluid warmer can rapidly warm and deliver up to 250 ml/min. If this equipment is not available another method is to warm crystalloid fluids with a microwave oven to 39°C.

The initial replacement fluid should be Ringer's lactate solution or normal saline. Hypertonic saline solutions are also currently under investigation for possible fluid replacement. Approximately 300 ml of crystalloid should be given for every estimated 100 ml of blood loss. In adults an initial bolus of one to two liters is given rapidly. The recommended dose for children is 20 ml/kg. Patients who do not respond or respond only transiently to the initial bolus will require blood transfusions as well as more crystalloid. All trauma patients must have blood drawn for type and crossmatch immediately on admission. Type-specific blood may be used in those patients who can not wait for a crossmatch. Those who present with exsanguinating hemorrhage will need O-negative blood immediately.

All trauma patients must be observed for early signs of shock. Those in shock must be aggressively monitored. In addition to blood pressure, heart rate, and neurological status, urine output and central venous pressure measurement can be useful. Adults should maintain a urinary output of at least 50 ml/hr. Pediatric patients should maintain at least 1 ml/kg/hr. Central venous pressure monitoring may also be helpful. Patients with shock need early surgical consultation and in many cases urgent surgical intervention.

Head Injuries

Cerebral injuries are a common cause of morbidity and mortality in the trauma patient. Because most rural hospitals do not have neurosurgeons on staff, the rural physician must be able to perform initial evaluation and emergency treatment of the head-injured patient. Management decisions are often made during telephone conversations with the neurosurgical consultant. The rural physician must be able to assess the patient accurately and communicate the findings to the consultant.

The head-injured patient is best assessed using the minineurological exam described by the Advanced Trauma Life Support Course (American College of Surgeons), which entails the following:

1. Assessment of the level of consciousness (LOC) using the Glasgow Coma Scale (GCS).
2. Pupillary function: size and reactivity to light.
3. Signs of lateralizing weakness.

The single most important part of the neurological exam is the level of consciousness, which is measured objectively by the Glasgow Coma Scale (Table 11.1). This should be assessed and carefully documented early in the course with repeated exams to watch closely for any change. A downward change in the GCS of 2 or more means the LOC has deteriorated. Evidence of deterioration is an important clinical finding that requires immediate intervention.

The management of the head-injured patient depends on the level of severity. For this purpose we will define four levels of severity: trivial, minor, moderate, and serious.

Table 11.1 The Glasgow Coma Scale

Eye opening		
	spontaneous	4
	to voice	3
	to pain	2
	none	1
Verbal response		
	oriented	5
	confused	4
	inappropriate words	3
	incomprehensible words	2
	none	1
Motor response		
	obeys commands	6
	localizes pain	5
	withdraws (pain)	4
	flexion (pain)	3
	extension (pain)	2
	none	1
Total Glasgow Coma Scale		15
Modification for verbal response in pediatric patients		
	social smile, fixes and follows	5
	cries, but consolable	4
	persistently irritable	3
	restless, agitated	2
	none	1

Trivial Head Injury

Glasgow Coma Scale 15
No loss of consciousness
Reliable history
Normal neurological exam

Management:

No CT scan or skull X rays needed (Masters, 1987)
Discharge with follow-up instructions

Minor Head Injury

Initial Glasgow Coma Scale 13-15

Management:

1. Oxygen: 10 L/min by nonrebreather mask
2. Evaluate cervical spine.
3. Obtain history. Duration of loss of consciousness.
4. Complete neurological exam including mental status.
5. Outpatient or Emergency Department observation for 6 hours if:
   a. Loss of consciousness less than 5 minutes
   b. Persistent headache or dizziness
   c. Normal neurological exam
6. Admit to Hospital for 24-hour observation and CT scan (if available) for any of the following:
   a. Loss of consciousness of greater than 5 minutes.
   b. Posttraumatic seizure
   c. Posttraumatic amnesia
   d. Alcohol or drug intoxication
   e. Progressive headache or vomiting
   f. Age less than 2
   g. Multisystem trauma
   h. Signs of basilar skull fracture
   i. Serious facial injury
   j. Possible depressed skull fracture
   k. Unreliable observer
   l. Suspected child abuse

If CT scanning of the brain is not available, a decision regarding transfer of the patient for this procedure should be made after discussion with a neurosurgeon. Skull X rays are of very little value except in the case of penetrating trauma or for suspected depressed skull fractures.

Moderate Head Injury

Initial Glasgow Coma Scale 9-13

Management:

1. Oxygen 10 L/min by nonrebreather mask
2. Control and evaluate the cervical spine
3. Monitor airway
4. History and neurological exam
5. CT scan and admit, or
6. Transfer to a trauma center for neurosurgical evaluation if there is no improvement in GCS or if CT scan is not available.

If the patient is restless or combative, consider causes such as hypotension, hypoxemia, hypoglycemia, or intoxication. If the patient does not have injuries that require immediate intubation, but control of the patient is a problem because the patient is agitated or combative, consider rapid sedation with a neuroleptic agent. Haloperidol is a safe and effective drug that will control a combative trauma patient. The dose is 5 mg IM or IV every 3-5 minutes until sedation is achieved. Benzodiazepines and opioids are not as effective for this purpose.

In the moderately severe head-injured patient who seems to be maintaining an adequate airway and requires transfer to another facility, consider the risk of deterioration during transfer and the possible need for airway control by intubation en route. This decision can be difficult and depends also on the duration of the transfer as well as the ability of the transport team to paralyze and intubate the patient en route should the patient deteriorate. A patient with an isolated head injury and a Glasgow Coma Scale of 10 or less should be intubated before transfer. Other multiple injuries might dictate intubation in a patient with a higher GCS.

Severe Head Injury

Initial Glasgow Coma Scale < 9

Management:

1. Evaluate and control cervical spine
2. Rapid sequence intubation
3. Hyperventilate to keep pCO_2 25-30 mm Hg

4. Prevent and treat hypotension
5. Unequal pupils or lateralizing motor exam, or downward change in GCS by 2 or more points:

    Mannitol 1 g/kg IV (500 ml of 20% Osmitrol = 100 g).

    Neurosurgical consultation by phone.
6. Seizures

    Diazepam 10 mg IV and diphenylhydantoin 18 mg/kg loading dose IV (rate < 50 mg/min).

    If no improvement, give phenobarbital 18 mg/kg IV loading dose.
7. Urgent transfer to a trauma center. Do not delay transfer for a CT scan if findings will not change the treatment at the rural hospital.

Amputations

Traumatic amputations of digits or extremities are not uncommon in rural areas. Amputations due to accidents on the farm are especially difficult because they often involve children, they result from shearing or crushing forces that cause much soft tissue damage, and wounds are heavily contaminated with bacteria. This section will address the approach and initial management of traumatic amputations.

The first objective is to assess the victim completely for other injuries and resuscitate and stabilize the patient as needed. More proximal amputations are often associated with other serious injuries. Seeing a patient with a dismembered extremity can create a strong emotional response causing the provider to focus on the injured extremity rather than adequately assessing and treating higher priority injuries such as airway difficulties or hypovolemic shock.

The rural physician is usually not the one to make the decision whether an amputated part will be replanted. This decision should be made by the surgeon and is often made in the operating room at the replantation center. The rural physician should not create false expectations. The patient should be told that he or she is being transferred to the replantation center in order to assess whether replantation is feasible and indicated.

The amputated part should always be sought. Replantation can be performed up to 4-6 hours after the accident with the amputated part at room temperature or up to 18 hours if cooled. In cases where replantation is not indicated, the amputated part may still be used for graft tissue.

Care of the Amputated Part: Complete Amputations

1. Rinse off any loose dirt or debris with sterile saline.
2. Wrap the part in a sterile towel that has been moistened with saline.
3. Place the wrapped part into a watertight plastic bag or container.
4. Place the plastic bag (or container) into an insulated cooling chest filled with ice water. Do not allow the amputated part to come into contact with ice directly. Do not use dry ice.

Care of the Amputated Part: Incomplete Amputations

1. Irrigate the wound with sterile saline.
2. Dress the wound with sterile dressings.
3. Apply a splint.
4. Surround the part with a bag of crushed ice.

Care of the Stump

1. Bleeding should be controlled using a soft, sterile pressure dressing. Control bleeding by direct pressure only. Do not use hemostats or tourniquets. In rare circumstances when bleeding cannot be controlled by pressure alone, a pneumatic tourniquet using a blood pressure cuff could be used.
2. Splint the extremity.
3. Start a large-bore IV in another extremity.
4. Give broad spectrum intravenous antibiotics.
5. Give tetanus toxoid or tetanus immune globulin if indicated.

Transferring the Patient

Trauma management requires getting the patient to definitive care as soon as possible after stabilization. If definitive care cannot be provided at the local hospital, then the patient will need to be transferred to a higher level facility. The criteria for transfer and a basic transfer checklist are included in Chapter 10. This is a decision requiring medical judgment and depends not only on the types of injuries but also on the resources available at the local hospital. Therefore, each rural hospital must develop its own transfer criteria based on locally available resources.

Research has proven that critically injured trauma patients have better outcomes when they are transferred to facilities that are prepared and dedicated to the care of the trauma patient. This will usually be a hospital that is designated or verified as a Level I or II trauma center by American College of Surgeons criteria.

The rural hospital should develop a relationship with a specific trauma center and establish transfer agreements with that facility. In some states these transfer criteria and relationships are mandated by law. It is important that the relationship with the trauma center be a two-way communication. The trauma center has the responsibility to participate in education and training of the rural hospital personnel. In addition, the trauma center should be willing to transfer patients back to the local community for long-term care and rehabilitation when appropriate.

The referring physician is responsible for maximal stabilization and transfer of the patient under the most optimal conditions. This may mean urgent surgical intervention or other intensive stabilization procedures.

Choosing the appropriate mode of transfer is essential. The level of care must not decline from one step to another as the patient moves through the trauma system. When available, the most appropriate mode of transport may be by helicopter with a transport team consisting of paramedics, critical care nurses, and in some cases a physician. A critical patient should not be transferred by ground ambulance under the care of EMTs with only basic-level skills. In cases where an advanced life-support or aeromedical service is not available, a nurse or physician from the rural hospital may decide to accompany the patient in transfer in order to continue to provide the highest available level of care.

Arrangements for transfer should be made early in the course of the evaluation and resuscitation of the patient. After performing the primary and secondary surveys, the physician will usually be able to decide whether or not the patient will require transfer. As soon as this decision has been made, the transport service should be summoned. In some protocols, a helicopter may be summoned to respond when the local hospital has been notified by the prehospital providers that a critical trauma patient has been encountered.

The patient should be transferred as soon as the injuries have been stabilized. Transfer should not be delayed for laboratory or radiologic procedures that will not change the immediate care. For example, a CT scan or peritoneal lavage should not be done at the rural hospital if it is not going to influence treatment prior to transfer.

Summary

Rural emergency physicians should be organized and prepared to provide basic emergency management of the four common conditions encountered in severely injured patients that we have discussed in this chapter. Relationships with a trauma center and transport service must be arranged in advance so that there will be no delay in transferring a patient who requires specialized services. Although critically injured patients may not be seen with frequency in rural emergency departments, the advance preparations can facilitate the necessary care and provide much professional satisfaction on the part of the physicians and other hospital personnel.

References

Campbell, J. E. (1988). *Basic trauma life support*. Englewood Cliffs, NJ: Prentice Hall.
Committee on Trauma of the American College of Surgeons. (1988). *Advanced life support textbook*. Chicago: American College of Surgeons.
Masters, S. J. (1987). Skull X-ray examination after head trauma. Recommendations by a multidisciplinary panel and validation study. *New England Journal of Medicine, 316*, 84-91.
Walls, R. M. (1992). The multiple trauma patient. In R. H. Dailey, R. D. Stewart, G. P. Young, & B. Simon (Eds.), *The airway: Emergency management*. St. Louis: Mosby Year Book.

Resource

American College of Surgeons
55 E. Erie Street
Chicago, IL 60611
(Advanced Trauma Life Support Course)

12
■ ■ ■

Treatment of Acute Myocardial Infarction With Thrombolytic Drugs in the Rural Hospital

ROY A. YAWN

Introduction

Intravenous thrombolytic therapy for eligible patients with acute myocardial infarction (MI) has become the standard of care in the United States. Every physician who attends such patients should have the expertise to administer thrombolytic agents promptly and appropriately. This is especially important in rural areas, where cardiac referral centers may be hours away even by helicopter, and sometimes inaccessible due to weather conditions. Even if the referral center is less than an hour away by ambulance, physicians should still be prepared to give thrombolytic agents, because the delay in therapy due to the transfer may diminish or negate any expected benefit.

The use of thrombolysis in acute MI has been shown to reduce short- and long-term mortality (GISSI, 1986; ISIS-2, 1988) by 25% to 50% and to decrease the incidence of serious arrhythmias (National Heart Foundation of Australia [NHF of Australia], 1988), left ventricular dysfunction (ISAM Study Group, 1986; White, Norrids, Brown et al., 1987), and congestive heart failure (Guerci, Gerstenblith, Brinker et al., 1987; NHF of Australia, 1988). The major risk of therapy is bleeding, especially intracranial bleeding, but the expected benefits of treatment outweigh the risks in the majority of patients (Grines & DeMaria, 1990; Tiefenbrunn & Ludbrook, 1989). Thrombolytic therapy in acute MI is underutilized in patients who are elderly; have a lower functional capacity; and a history of previous MI, hypertension, angina, or diabetes (Pfeffer, Moye, Braunwald et al., 1991). A major problem currently is that many physicians decline to administer thrombolytic drugs because of concern about bleeding, especially in the elderly (Gurwitz, Goldberg, & Gore, 1991). Rural physicians may also have concerns about access to blood products if needed, coronary care unit personnel and their experience, and medical backup in case of complications or a necessary absence of the treating physician. Nevertheless, physicians must not shirk the responsibility of giving thrombolytic drugs because of fear of complications.

One extra life will be saved for each 20 to 25 acute MI patients treated with thrombolytics (ISIS-2, 1988; GISSI-2, 1990a, 1990b). The incidence of stroke in acute MI is about 1%, whether treated with thrombolytics or not, with about half of those being fatal (Maggioni, Franzosa, Santoro et al., 1992). Thus, in treating 200 patients one would potentially save 8 to 10 lives, with about 1 death from stroke. A small hospital treating 20 to 25 patients with acute MI per year would be saving one life per year, and would see about one fatal stroke associated with MI in 8 to 10 years.

Selection of Patients

Inclusion and exclusion criteria for patients eligible for thrombolysis are outlined in Table 12.1. Patients should have symptoms consistent with acute MI, including typical chest pain, dyspnea, diaphoresis, nausea, or vomiting; and they must have electrocardiographic evidence of an acute MI, defined as ST segment elevation of one or more millimeters in at least two limb leads, or two or more millimeters in at least two precordial leads (Simoons, 1989). In addition, symptoms should have been present for 6 hours or less. There may be some benefit from thrombolysis if given more than 6 hours after the onset of symptoms (ISIS-2, 1988); and if a patient is continuing to have chest pain for more than 6 hours, thrombolysis may still be warranted. This is especially pertinent if a large anterior infarct is present.

Absolute contraindications for thrombolytic therapy are active internal bleeding and previous cerebrovascular events including stroke or transient cerebral ischemia (ISIS-2, 1988; Simoons, 1989).

Table 12.1 Contraindications for Thrombolytic Therapy

Absolute Contraindications

> Active gastrointestinal bleeding or ulcer
> History of stroke or transient cerebral ischemia

Relative Contraindications

> Recent major trauma, especially head trauma
> Noncompressible vascular punctures
> Pregnancy or recent obstetrical delivery
> History of bleeding disorder
> Major surgery in the last 3-6 months
> Severe uncontrolled or malignant hypertension
> Allergy to streptokinase or APSAC or administration within 6 months
> Prolonged cardiopulmonary resuscitation (> 1 min)
> Proliferative diabetic retinopathy

Additional contraindications include major surgery or trauma within the past 6 months, brain surgery or tumor, pregnancy, bleeding disorders, proliferative diabetic retinopathy, recent noncompressible vascular puncture, prolonged cardiopulmonary resuscitation (more than 1 minute), and uncontrolled hypertension. If the blood pressure is more than 180/100, it is preferable to lower the pressure with intravenous nitroglycerin or nitroprusside before initiating thrombolysis.

Except for active bleeding, the listed contraindications must be considered to be theoretical. For example, there are no large studies that show that the actual risk of intracranial bleeding from thrombolysis is increased in patients with previous stroke. Indeed, studies are currently under way to evaluate the use of thrombolytic agents in acute stroke syndromes; and the preliminary data indicate no increased risk of cerebral hemorrhage (Mori, Yoneda, Ohksawa et al., 1991). In ISIS-3 (1992), 3.6% of the randomized patients had a history of stroke, and 8.6% had a previous gastrointestinal bleed or ulcer. Even patients on oral anticoagulants may receive thrombolytic agents, as is being done in the GUSTO study (discussed below).

When considering the use of thrombolytic drugs, the physician must try to balance the benefits and risks for the patient in question. For the patient who is relatively young and otherwise healthy, and who presents to the hospital soon after suffering a large anterior infarction, the potential benefits are large; and the physician should make every effort to administer thrombolytic agents. However, if the patient is old and frail, with multisystem diseases, and has a small uncomplicated inferior infarction, thrombolysis is unlikely to lead to much benefit.

Age alone is not a contraindication to thrombolysis, but because complications increase with age and the benefits are less well defined, therapy should be individualized (Gurwitz et al., 1991). In the ISIS-2 (1988) study, mortality after acute MI in patients over 70 treated with streptokinase (SK) and aspirin was 15.8%, versus 23.8% in the placebo group. Treatment with SK or anisoylated plasminogen-streptokinase activator (APSAC) within 6 months or a history of a severe allergic reaction are considered contraindications to re-treatment with the same agent. In these cases tissue thromboplastin activator (tPA) can be considered.

Informed Consent

The question of whether to require a formal signed consent for thrombolytic therapy frequently arises. Because this is now standard therapy, a signed consent form is probably not necessary. Also, obtaining truly informed consent is problematic in a patient with a life threatening illness who is having pain and who may have received drugs that impair the mental status. The possibility of bleeding complications, including cerebral hemorrhage, should be explained to the patient and family.

Evaluation Before Administering
Thrombolytic Agents

Sample orders are outlined in Table 12.2. Once the diagnosis of acute MI has been made, the laboratory studies should be ordered promptly and drawn at once; further venipunctures must be kept to the minimum. The results of the studies do not have to be completed before starting therapy. If the clinical assessment does not suggest other problems or contraindications, it is reasonable to proceed with thrombolysis before all results are available.

Table 12.2 Sample Protocol for Administration of Streptokinase

1. Diagnosis of acute MI by clinical assessment and EKG

2. Lab: CBC, platelet count, PT, PTT, CPK, CPK-MB, Na, K, BUN, creatinine, glucose
   X ray: obtain a portable chest X ray, but do not delay the SK infusion

3. Review medical history for contraindications

4. Administer 162 mg of chewable aspirin

5. Establish 2 or 3 IV sites (18-gauge needles) with IV pumps

6. Administer analgesics, fluids, sublingual or IV nitroglycerine as needed

7. Baseline neurologic check

8. Streptokinase 1.5 million units by IV pump over 60 minutes

9. Heparin 5,000 U IV bolus simultaneously with the start of the SK infusion OR after the SK infusion is completed

10. Heparin 1,000-1,200 U per hour by IV infusion

11. After the SK infusion, if there is no contraindication:
    Atenolol 5 MG IV over 5 min; repeat in 15 min (total IV dose 10 mg)
    Atenolol 50 mg orally 10 min after the last IV dose and daily thereafter

12. PTT 6 hours after starting heparin. Adjust PTT to 1.5-2.0 times the control level, using a heparin nomogram

13. Assess for resolution of chest pain, decreased ST segment elevation, improved hemodynamics, stable neurologic status

14. Observe for reperfusion arrhythmias. PVCs and idioventricular rhythm ("slow V. tach.") without hemodynamic compromise do not require treatment.

15. Indications for discontinuation of thrombolytic therapy: allergic reactions (anaphylaxis, bronchospasm, rash, hypotension not controlled by leg elevation or fluid bolus); development of significant hemorrhage or change in neurologic status

In large hospitals, thrombolytic agents are frequently administered in the emergency department. In a small rural hospital, it may be more practical to transfer the patient to the coronary care unit while the infusions are being mixed, because the most experienced personnel will most likely be coronary care unit nurses. The transfer should result in minimal, if any, delay in starting therapy in this case.

Choice of Thrombolytic Agent

The drug of choice at the time of this writing is clearly strepto-kinase. Although tPA may result in earlier and more frequent coro-nary patency (Marder & Sherry, 1988), its use also entails a higher risk of reocclusion, and a slight excess of strokes. Furthermore, mortality and bleeding complications are not significantly different from those of SK (GISSI-2, 1990a; ISIS-3, 1992). Finally, the cost of SK is only about one-tenth the cost of tPA. If your hospital treats a substantial number of Medicare patients with acute MI, you may find that the reimbursement does not cover hospital costs, even without thrombolytic agents.

Currently under way is the GUSTO study (Global Utilization of Streptokinase and tPA for Occluded Coronary Arteries), involving 40,000 patients, which directly compares the efficacy of strepto-kinase, tPA, and the combination of SK and tPA. This study may shed some additional light on which agent, if either, is superior. At this time, however, it is appropriate and acceptable practice to use streptokinase routinely, and to reserve tPA for patients who are allergic to SK, who have received SK within 6 months, or who may need a second dose of thrombolytics because of recurrent chest pain with ST elevation.

Method of Administration

The standard dose of SK is 1.5 million units administered by intra-venous infusion over 60 minutes. Establish two or three IV sites if possible, for the administration of SK as well as analgesics, fluids, lidocaine, or other indicated drugs. Usually 45 to 60 minutes are re-quired to obtain evidence of reperfusion, such as decreased chest pain, decrease in ST segment elevation, and reperfusion arrhythmias.

Intravenous infusion of SK may result in hypotension in 10% of treated patients, compared to 2% in patients given a placebo (ISIS-2, 1988). This should be treated with leg elevation and infusion of normal saline. If the hypotension persists, the rate of infusion of SK may be decreased and pressor agents may be needed. The hypoten-sion may also be the result of the myocardial damage rather than due to SK, and finishing the SK infusion is in the best interest of the patient in this case.

Adjunctive Therapy

The addition of aspirin to SK clearly results in greater survival (ISIS-2, 1988) for patients with acute MI. Our practice is to give two 81 mg chewable aspirin tablets to the patient at the start of the SK infusion, and to continue a dose of 81 mg daily and indefinitely in the absence of contraindications.

Beta-blockers have been shown to independently reduce mortality in acute MI (Yusef, Peto, Lewis, Collins, & Sleight, 1985; ISIS-1, 1986). In the absence of hypotension, bradycardia, or congestive heart failure, atenolol or metoprolol should be given intravenously after the SK infusion is completed. Atenolol is given as 5 mg IV over 5 minutes in two doses 15 minutes apart (total IV dose 10 mg), then 50 mg orally 10 minutes after the last IV dose and daily thereafter. Metoprolol can be given as three IV boluses of 5 mg 2 minutes apart for a total dose of 15 mg if tolerated, followed by 50 mg orally every 6 hours for 24 hours, then 50-100 mg each day.

In the United States, heparin is usually given along with or after the SK infusion to reduce the incidence of coronary reocclusion and to prevent thrombotic events. A bolus of 5,000 units may be given at the start of the SK infusion, or at the end, followed by an intravenous infusion of 1,000-1,200 units per hour. A partial thromboplastin time (PTT) should be checked about 6 hours after the initiation of SK and heparin, and the heparin dose should be adjusted to maintain a PTT of 1.5-2.0 times the control value. The use of a heparin nomogram may help to maintain the PTT in a therapeutic range (Cruickshank, Levine, Hirsch, Roberts, & Siguenza, 1991). Continue the intravenous heparin for a minimum of 48 hours.

In Europe, the use of heparin after SK is not considered mandatory, and some physicians either do not administer heparin or give it subcutaneously as 12,500 units every 12 hours. The GUSTO study treated a group with subcutaneous heparin, and the physician should look for the publication of these results for further guidance about the use of heparin after SK infusion for treatment of acute MI.

Intravenous nitroglycerin can be given simultaneously with SK (though not through the same intravenous tubing) if it is needed for control of continued chest pain, congestive heart failure, or hypertension. Start with an infusion of 5 micrograms per minute and adjust the dose about every 10 minutes according to the clinical situation.

If the patient is not a candidate for thrombolytic therapy but has clearly suffered an acute MI, strongly consider giving aspirin, heparin, beta-blockers, and intravenous nitroglycerin. These agents will improve the patient's chance of survival even if thrombolysis is not undertaken. Giving intravenous steroids before starting SK infusions to prevent allergic reactions is no longer a standard practice. Likewise, prophylactic administration of lidocaine is usually not carried out.

Complications

The most feared complication of thrombolytic therapy is intracranial hemorrhage. The incidence of all strokes in patients receiving thrombolytic agents for acute MI is about 1% (GISSI-2, 1990a; ISIS-3, 1992; Maggioni et al., 1992), which is about the same rate as in the pre-thrombolytic era, when most strokes were presumed to be thrombotic rather than hemorrhagic (Tiefenbrunn & Ludbrook, 1989). About one half of strokes associated with thrombolysis are hemorrhagic. The mortality from stroke of all causes in the ISIS-2 study was 0.3%, which was similar to the death rate from stroke in the control group, which did not receive thrombolytic therapy. Although a stroke in a patient with acute MI may be disastrous, even when thrombolysis has been withheld, large amounts of data indicate that the risk of dying of acute MI is much larger than the risk of death from stroke, and that thrombolytic therapy can reduce the mortality rate by 25% to 50%.

If there is any evidence of new neurologic symptoms or stroke in a patient who is receiving or has received thrombolytic agents, these agents and heparin should be stopped. If heparin has been administered within 4 hours of bleeding, protamine sulfate should be considered. It may be necessary to give cryoprecipitate or fresh frozen plasma to normalize coagulation parameters. A computed tomographic (CT) scan of the brain should be performed to ascertain the nature of the stroke. If CT scanning is not available in the treating institution, transfer to another center may be necessary. A detailed analysis of bleeding during thrombolytic therapy and an algorithm for treatment has been published (Sane, Califf, Topol et al., 1989).

Bleeding from sites other than the brain can be managed by discontinuing thrombolytic agents and anticoagulant therapy, and supporting the patient with fresh frozen plasma and packed red blood cells as necessary. About 3 patients per 1,000 treated with thrombolytic agents will require transfusions because of hemorrhage (ISIS-2, 1988).

Follow-Up Care

If the patient obtains relief of chest pain after thrombolysis, vital signs are stable, and there is no sign of congestive heart failure or recurrent angina, care can be advanced according to the usual coronary care unit protocol. In the absence of complications after acute MI treated with thrombolytic agents, coronary angiography is no longer considered necessary in every patient. If there are no further complications or problems during the remainder of the hospital stay, a low-level treadmill stress test can be done at discharge or shortly thereafter to assess functional capacity and the presence or absence of exercise-induced ischemia. The absence of ischemic changes and a reasonable exercise capacity shown by treadmill testing indicates that the patient can be treated medically and that invasive procedures are not required.

If the patient experiences recurrent chest pain, signs of congestive heart failure, or life-threatening arrhythmias, referral to a cardiology center should be considered. Details of risk stratification and management after acute MI are beyond the scope of this chapter and are thoroughly discussed in the review by Krone (1992).

Summary

Thrombolytic therapy is the treatment of choice in acute MI patients meeting basic criteria and having no active bleeding. Physicians should be aggressive in administering thrombolytic drugs in these situations, and must not view long lists of relative contraindications as excuses to avoid these agents. Bleeding complications are generally infrequent and are managed by discontinuing the thrombolytic drug and supporting with transfusions as necessary. The risk of stroke has not changed in the thrombolytic era, and the risk of death from acute MI and its complications far exceeds the risk of death from stroke.

References

Cruickshank, M. K., Levine, M. N., Hirsch, H., Roberts, R., & Siguenza, M. (1991). A standard nomogram for the management of heparin therapy. *Archives of Internal Medicine, 151,* 333-337.

GISSI (Gruppo Italiana per lo Studio della Streptochinasi nell'Infarto Miocardico). (1986). Effectiveness of intravenous thrombolytic treatment in acute myocardial infarction. *Lancet, 1,* 397-402.

GISSI-2 (Gruppo Italiana per lo Studio della Streptochinasi nell'Infarto Miocardico). (1990a). A factorial randomised trial of alteplase versus streptokinase and heparin versus no heparin among 12,490 patients with acute myocardial infarction. *Lancet, 336,* 65-70.

GISSI-2 (Gruppo Italiana per lo Studio della Streptochinasi nell'Infarto Miocardico). (1990b). In-hospital mortality and clinical course of 20,891 patients with suspected acute myocardial infarction randomised between alteplase and streptokinase with or without heparin. *Lancet, 336,* 71-75.

Grines, C. L., & DeMaria, A. N. (1990). Optimal utilization of thrombolytic therapy for acute myocardial infarction: Concepts and controversies. *Journal of American College of Cardiology, 16,* 223-231.

Guerci, A. D., Gerstenblith, G., Brinker, J., et al. (1987). A randomized trial of intravenous tissue plasminogen activator for acute myocardial infarction with subsequent randomization to elective coronary angiography. *New England Journal of Medicine, 317,* 1613-1618.

Gurwitz, J. H., Goldberg, R. J., & Gore, J. M. (1991). Coronary thrombolysis for the elderly? *Journal of the American Medical Association, 265,* 1720-1723.

ISAM Study Group. (1986). A prospective trial of intravenous streptokinase in acute myocardial infarction. Mortality, morbidity and infarct size at 21 days. *New England Journal of Medicine, 314,* 1465-1471.

ISIS-1 (First International Study of Infarct Survival) Collaborative Group. (1986). Randomized trial of intravenous atenolol among 16,027 cases of suspected acute myocardial infarction. *Lancet, 2,* 57-65.

ISIS-2 (Second International Study of Infarct Survival) Collaborative Group. (1988). Randomized trial of intravenous streptokinase, oral aspirin, both, or neither among 17,187 cases of suspected acute myocardial infarction. *Lancet, 2,* 349-360.

ISIS-3 (Third International Study of Infarct Survival) Collaborative Group. (1992). A randomized comparison of streptokinase vs tissue plasminogen activator vs anistreplase and of aspirin vs heparin alone among 41,299 cases of suspected acute myocardial infarction. *Lancet, 399,* 753-770.

Krone, R. J. (1992). The role of risk stratification in the early management of a myocardial infarction. *Annals of Internal Medicine, 116,* 223-237.

Maggioni, A. P., Franzosa, M. A., Santoro, E., et al. (1992). The risk of stroke in patients with acute myocardial infarction after thrombolytic and antithrombotic treatment. *New England Journal of Medicine, 327*, 1-6.

Marder, V. J., & Sherry S. (1988). Thrombolytic therapy: Current status (Parts 1 and 2). *New England Journal of Medicine, 318*, 1512-1520, 1585-1595.

Mori, E., Yoneda, Y., Ohksawa, S., et al. (1991). Double-blind placebo-controlled trial of recombinant tissue plasminogen activator (tPA) in acute carotid stroke [Abstract]. *Neurology, 41*(Suppl. 1), 347.

National Heart Foundation of Australia Coronary Thrombolysis Group (NHF of Australia). (1988). Coronary thrombolysis and myocardial salvage by tissue plasminogen activator given up to 4 hours after onset of myocardial infarction. *Lancet, 1*, 203-207.

Pfeffer, M, A., Moye, L. A., Braunwald, E., et al. (1991). Selection bias in the use of thrombolytic therapy in acute myocardial infarction. *Journal of the American Medical Association, 266*, 528-532.

Sane, D. C., Califf, R. M., Topol, E. J., et al. (1989). Bleeding during thrombolytic therapy for acute myocardial infarction: Mechanisms and management. *Annals of Internal Medicine, 111*, 1010-1022.

Simoons, M. L. (1989). Thrombolytic therapy in acute myocardial infarction. *Annual Review of Medicine, 40*, 181-200.

Tiefenbrunn, A. J., & Ludbrook, P. A. (1989). Coronary thrombolysis: It's worth the risk. *Journal of the American Medical Association, 261*, 2107-2108.

White, H. D., Norrids, R., Brown, M. A., et al. (1987). Effect of intravenous streptokinase on left ventricular function and early survival after acute myocardial infarction. *New England Journal of Medicine, 317*, 850-855.

Yusef, S., Peto, R., Lewis, J., Collins, R., & Sleight, P. (1985). Beta blockade during and after myocardial infarction: An overview of the randomized trials. *Progress in Cardiovascular Disease, 27*, 335-371.

13
■ ■ ■

Women's Health Issues

CHERI L. OLSON

Introduction

The decade of the 1990s is the decade of women's health. An explosion of research, policy, and patient demand are driving care providers to be aware, knowledgeable, and sensitive to women's health issues. Many women today are seeking to be partners in health care, while taking an increased responsibility for their own bodies. This chapter will cover some of the women's health problems commonly encountered in rural practice.

Prevention

Frequent visits of women in their reproductive years for Pap tests, prenatal care, and contraceptive advice and prescriptions allow the physician an excellent opportunity to provide longitudinal care and education. It is never too early or too late to educate women about clinical breast examination, osteoporosis, sexually transmitted diseases, and mammography.

Pap Tests

Pap tests and pelvic examinations should begin with the beginning of sexual activity or at age 18. A visit for a Pap test should include the clinical breast examination, education about breast self-

examination (BSE), and a review of the patient's history as well as
the pelvic examination.

Recent concern has focused on the quality and frequency of Pap
tests. Although frequency may be open to individualization, quality is not. A properly performed Pap test contains the following
elements:

1. Visualization of the cervix with a warmed speculum.
2. Minimal removal of mucus obscuring the cervix.
3. Sampling of the endocervix with a cytology brush by inserting the
   brush into the cervix and rotating approximately 180 degrees (omit if
   patient is pregnant).
4. Smear the cytology brush on one half of a glass slide with a one-pass
   rolling movement.
5. Sample the ectocervix with wooden or plastic spatula.
6. Smear the spatula sample on the other half of the slide.

The Abnormal Pap Test

The Pap test report should be viewed as a medical consultation
between pathologist and practitioner. Pap test classifications vary
widely, but there is a growing consensus that the "class" system
(I-V) is inadequate. The four commonly used systems for reporting
Pap test results and their relationships are shown in Figure 13.1.

All patients with cervical dysplasia should undergo colposcopy.
Patients with "atypia" or "inflammation" should probably have
colposcopy because one third of these will have dysplasia. Some
experts believe that treating an identifiable cervical or vaginal path-
ogen when the Pap test shows "inflammation" and repeating the
Pap test in 3 months may be an alternative. If "inflammation" persists at 3 months, colposcopy is performed. Other indications for
colposcopy are listed in Table 13.1.

Rural physicians must become skilled in colposcopy and in the
treatment of cervical pathology or find a consultant who has these
skills. Colposcopic skills would be highly valued in a rural practice
because patient compliance is improved by evaluation, treatment,
and follow-up by her personal physician.

Class System	World Health Organization System	Cervical Intraepithelial Neoplasia System	Bethesda System
I	Normal	Normal	Within normal limits
II	Inflammation		Other infection, reactive, and reparative
III	Dysplasia Mild Moderate Severe	 CIN-1 CIN-2	Squamous intra-epithelial lesions Low grade High grade
IV	Carcinoma in situ	CIN-3	
V	Invasive squamous cell carcinoma Adenocarcinoma	Invasive squamous carcinoma Adenocarcinoma	Squamous cell carcinoma Adenocarcinoma

Figure 13.1. Cytopathology Reporting Systems for Pap Tests

Screening for Breast Cancer

Implementation of current screening recommendations has been shown to decrease breast cancer mortality by 25%. Breast cancer screening includes:

1. Monthly breast self-examination.
2. Annual physician/practitioner breast examination.
3. Mammography at age-appropriate intervals:
     age 35-39: a "baseline" screening mammogram.
     age 40-49: every 2 years if low risk.
     age 50-75: yearly.
     age > 75: every 2 years.

Table 13.1 Indications for Colposcopy

Dysplasia (mild, moderate, or severe)
Squamous cell carcinoma
Adenocarcinoma
Visible cervical abnormality (even if the Pap test is normal)
Human papillomavirus infection (cervical or external genitalia)
Persistent inflammation
Atypia
High risk for cervical dysplasia (other sexually transmitted diseases, herpes
  simplex virus infection, HIV infection, smoking)

The presence of risk factors for the development of breast cancer should increase the recommended frequency of mammography screening and physician breast exam to annually after age 40. The most significant risk factors for breast cancer are family history of breast cancer, early age at menarche, late age at the birth of the first child (> 30 years), nulliparity, and late age at menopause.

The Breast Lump

There is almost no event so frightening to a woman as finding a lump in her breast. Speedy diagnostic evaluation is critical due to the immense anxiety associated with the discovery of a lump. The rural physician may have to exert extra effort to minimize diagnostic delay.

Any breast lump must be evaluated, regardless of whether the mammogram is normal or abnormal. This evaluation may include a limited period of observation, needle aspiration, excision, or referral to a breast specialist. A negative or normal mammogram, when a lump is present, is not necessarily reassuring, because mammography will miss breast cancers 10%-15% of the time.

A careful history, physical examination, and risk assessment will help select those women who need surgical evaluation rather than observation by their physicians. One approach to the evaluation of breast lumps, presented in Figure 13.2, is based on needle aspiration of any lump on the initial office visit. This is especially important in younger women, and can provide quick reassurance when mammography is not immediately available. In settings where mammo-

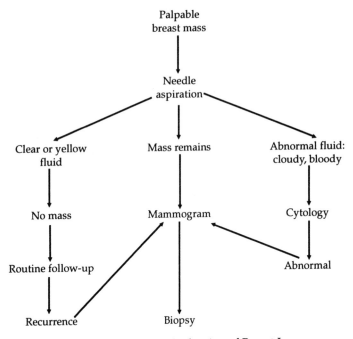

Figure 13.2. An Algorithm for the Evaluation of Breast Lumps

graphy is available on-site, many physicians would prefer X-ray evaluation before needle aspiration.

The technique of needle aspiration is easy, and can be both diagnostic and therapeutic. The skin is infiltrated with a small amount of 1% lidocaine. The lesion should be firmly held with one hand while a 20 or 21 gauge needle attached to a 10 ml syringe held with continuous suction is passed through the lesion. The material obtained is smeared on a slide. Clear fluid is unlikely to be found in malignant lesions. Cloudy or bloody fluid should be sent for cytological examination.

Multiple options for treatment of breast cancer exist and are constantly changing. The current medical literature and a surgical oncology specialist should be consulted regularly to assure appropriate referrals.

Table 13.2 Annual Failure Rates of Contraceptive Methods

	Typical Failure Rate (percentage)	Optimal Use Failure Rate (percentage)
Natural Family Planning	20	10
Diaphragm	18	3
Condom	10	3
Cervical Cap	18	3
Spermicidal Foam/Suppository	20-25	3
Sponge: parous women	28	9
Sponge: nulliparous women	18	6
IUD	3-5	2
Oral Contraceptives	4-10	0.3
Norplant	0.2	0.2
Sterilization-Tubal Ligation	0.4	0.2

Contraception

The decision to use a contraceptive method will be based on many factors including the patient's age, general health, weight, plans for further children, pregnancy spacing, smoking, parity, gynecologic history, breast cancer history, thromboembolic disease history, finances, and motivation. Table 13.2 shows typical failure rates and "optimal use" failure rates for common contraceptive methods.

A variety of nonhormonal and hormonal contraceptive methods exist. Many patients prefer nonhormonal methods, especially if the need for contraception is infrequent or if personal beliefs or medical risks prohibit hormone use.

Barrier Methods

Barrier methods include the diaphragm, cervical cap, sponge, and condoms. In well-motivated patients, pregnancy rates can be acceptably low. There are few contraindications to the use of barrier methods other than allergy to spermicides or latex and noncompliance. Nonlatex condoms do not provide adequate protection from sexually transmitted diseases. Spermicide containing nonoxynol-9 adds extra protection. Women may have an increased risk of urinary tract infections when using the diaphragm.

Natural Family Planning (NFP)

Highly motivated women with fairly regular cycles may be good candidates for NFP. Techniques involve assessing several parameters of fertility, such as cervical mucus, basal body temperature, and cervical consistency, and avoiding intercourse at fertile times if pregnancy is not desired. Classes are available through many Catholic churches.

Intrauterine device (IUD)

An IUD may be an excellent choice for a patient who wants efficacious birth control, without hormonal effect, using a noncoitus-related contraceptive. Intrauterine devices probably work locally at the uterine level to interfere with sperm transport, fertilization, and implementation. Only two IUDs are currently available. One contains progestin and must be replaced every 12 months; the other contains copper and does not require replacement for at least 6 years.

Because IUD users have an increased risk of developing pelvic inflammatory disease (PID) and ectopic pregnancy, IUDs should be used cautiously in nulliparous women and women in nonmonogamous relationships. A history of PID or ectopic pregnancy is a contraindication to use of an IUD. Insertion is relatively simple, and should be done within 2 days of the end of a normal menstrual period.

Oral Contraceptives

Today's oral contraceptives (OCs) are very effective, easily reversible, and quite safe. However, misperceptions about the safety of OCs persist. Over the past 20 years, the estrogen and progestin content of OCs has been reduced significantly, which has reduced the side-effect profile. Mild side effects include menstrual irregularity, weight gain, acne, and breast tenderness. More serious complications such as migraine, stroke, hypertension, and thrombophlebitis have been decreased by the lower dose OC formulations. In addi-

Table 13.3 Health Benefits of Oral Contraceptives

Fewer ovarian cysts
Decreased endometrial cancer
Decreased ovarian cancer
Decreased benign breast disease
Decreased pelvic inflammatory disease
Regular menses and less dysfunctional uterine bleeding
Less menorrhagia and anemia
Less dysmenorrhea
Fewer ectopic pregnancies
Decreased fibroids
Cardiovascular protective effect

tion to contraception, OCs have several noncontraceptive benefits (Table 13.3). Despite their many benefits and established safety, not every woman will be a candidate for OCs (Table 13.4).

Appropriate patient education about "nuisance" side effects, the mechanics of taking the pill, and other medication interactions will enhance compliance with OC use. Patient handouts regarding start dates, spotting, missed pills, and other details may be particularly helpful. Family planning clinics have excellent patient education materials regarding contraception.

Progestin Implants

The Norplant System is a new method of contraception introduced in the United States in January 1991. Clinical trials in more than 400,000 women in the United States and other countries have shown the levonorgestrel implants to be safe, well-tolerated, extremely effective, and easily reversible. Six silastic tubes, each containing 36 milligrams of levonorgestrel, are placed subdermally on the inside of the upper arm. Insertion under local anesthesia is an office procedure requiring 15-30 minutes. A trocar is used to insert the implants through a 2-millimeter incision. If inserted within the first 7 days after the onset of menses, contraception is effective within 24 hours and lasts for 5 years. If implanted later in the menstrual cycle, the contraceptive effect can be delayed until the next cycle.

Levonorgestrel implants appear to work in several ways. Ovulation is inhibited in about 50% of cycles. Cervical mucus is thickened,

Table 13.4 Contraindications to Oral Contraceptive Use

Absolute
    History of venous or arterial thrombosis
    Severe hypertension (in most cases)
    Poorly controlled diabetes (in most cases)
    Known/suspected breast cancer
    Estrogen-dependent neoplasia
    Pregnancy
    Undiagnosed genital bleeding
    History of a liver tumor or current impaired liver function
    Smoker aged 35 or greater (> 15 cig/d)

Relative ("Red Flag")
    Mild hypertension
    Morbid obesity
    Migraine headache
    Family history of early vascular disease

thus resisting sperm penetration. Fertility returns quickly after removal, and 80% to 90% of women are successful in achieving pregnancy within 1 year.

Careful patient counseling and selection are vital to physician and patient acceptance of the Norplant System. Disadvantages of implants include the need for surgical insertion and removal, the cost of more than $500 (in 1992), the androgenic side effects, and irregular, unpredictable bleeding. The major advantage is the provision of extremely effective, noncoitus-related, reversible contraception. With careful counseling, instruction, and patient selection, unplanned removals can be kept to a minimum. A 3-month trial of a progestin-only OC ("mini-pill") may be considered before insertion of implants. Removal of implants will take about 30 to 60 minutes.

Norplant System counseling and insertion are relatively simple and easily learned skills. Many conferences are offering workshops to train physicians to insert implants. This skill is a valuable one for rural family physicians.

Depo-Provera

Depo-Provera has recently been approved for contraceptive use. A dose of 150 milligrams is given intramuscularly during the first 5 days of menses and every 3 months thereafter. Advantages include the use of a progestin-only contraceptive, no regular maintenance by the patient except periodic visits to the physician, and provider-administered medication. Disadvantages are irregular breakthrough bleeding, quarterly intramuscular injections, and slow reversibility.

Vaginitis

Some physicians estimate that as many as 50% of all gynecologic office visits are for evaluation of vaginitis. Symptoms may vary from none to disabling. Routine treatment without vaginal and pelvic examinations and simple laboratory tests is to be avoided in most cases. In general, all testing necessary to diagnose vaginitis can be done in the rural physician's office. The most common types of vaginitis with distinguishing characteristics and treatment are listed in Figure 13.3.

Sexually Transmitted Diseases

Each year, at least 12 million cases of sexually transmitted diseases (STDs) occur in the United States, primarily in 15- to 30-year-olds. This number probably underestimates the true magnitude of the problem, because underreporting is common. Morbidity includes infertility, pelvic inflammatory disease, ectopic pregnancy, and increased perinatal morbidity and mortality. This section will deal with some STDs commonly seen in rural practice. Infection with the human immunodeficiency virus (HIV) is discussed in another chapter in this book. All persons found to have one STD should be evaluated for others, that is, inspection for genital warts, a Pap test for cervical dysplasia, a serologic test for syphilis, and testing (with informed consent) for HIV. Confidentiality, especially in treating adolescents, is important to remember in rural practices, where few patients are not known by someone on the office staff.

Chlamydia

For the past 20 years, chlamydia has been the leading cause of STDs in the United States. Chlamydia continues to spread rapidly

Diagnosis	Bacterial Vaginosis	Monilial Vaginitis	Trichomonas Vaginitis	Atrophic Vaginitis
Age	sexually active	all ages	sexually active	peri or post menopausal
Appearance of discharge	homogenous, gray-white discharge; wipes easily off vaginal walls	thick, curdy, white, "cottage cheese"	green, frothy, copious fluid	minimal to no fluid
Appearance of cervix and vagina	often normal except for discharge	adherent curdy discharge; cervix normal	cervix shows pathognomonic "strawberry" punctation	dry, pale tissue; superficial erosions
Vaginal pH	> 4.5	4.0 - 4.5	4.0 - 4.5	5.5 - 7
Wet prep/KOH	"clue" cells	budding yeast; hyphae	motile protozoans	nonspecific
Other diagnostic tests	"whiff" test: fishy odor of vaginal discharge when treated with 10% KOH			vaginal smear fixed to slide with Pap fixative: pathology report: 80-20-0 basal, intermediate, superficial versus estrogenized vagina 0-20-80
Treatment	Metronidazole 500 mg p.o. BID for 7 days Clindamycin 150 mg p.o. BID for 7 days Metronidazole vaginal gel 1 applicator BID for 5 days	Teraconazole 0.4% cream per vagina for 3 days Other imidazoles, e.g., miconazole	metronidazole 250 mg p.o. TID for 5 days Treat sexual partner	Estrogen by any route Nonhormonal moisturizing cream

Figure 13.3 Common Vaginal Infactions

Table 13.5 History and Physical Risk Factors for Chlamydia Infection

Mucopurulent cervicitis
History of sexually transmitted diseases
Abnormal bleeding after sexual intercourse
Partner with history of nongonococcal urethritis
Multiple sexual partners
Abnormal vaginal or cervical discharge
No contraceptive or nonbarrier contraceptive use
New sexual partner (< 2 months)
Young women 18-35 (especially < 20)
Dysuria
Dyspareunia

because at least 75% of infected women will remain asymptomatic. Chlamydial infections are estimated to cause 250,000 cases of PID, 30,000 cases of infertility, and 10,000 cases of ectopic pregnancy per year in the United States. Because of the high incidence of asymptomatic infections, the rural physician must identify, test, and treat high-risk patients. Common risk factors are listed in Table 13.5.

Chlamydia is not an easy organism to identify. Culture is the "gold standard" but is expensive, difficult to interpret, performed primarily at large urban centers, and takes 24-48 hours to complete. A variety of antigen detection techniques and assays have been developed that are rapid and fairly accurate. Treatment of chlamydia is simple. Doxycycline, 100 milligrams twice daily, or tetracycline, 500 milligrams twice daily, for 7 days is preferred. For pregnant patients or those allergic to tetracyclines, erythromycin 500 milligrams four times daily for 7 days is used. The Centers for Disease Control (CDC) guidelines currently call for treating the woman with chlamydia for gonorrhea as well because of the high incidence of concurrent disease.

Recently azithromycin 1 gram orally as a single dose has been shown to be effective for chlamydia. Ideally, sexual partners should be examined and treated accordingly, but empiric treatment of partners may be necessary.

Human Papilloma Virus

Human papilloma virus (HPV) causes genital warts and is today the most common viral STD. About 5%-30% of all women have been

shown to have HPV. Some studies have revealed that up to 75% of
college women are infected with HPV. HPV infection is associated
with cervical dysplasia and carcinoma of the cervix. External condylomata can be treated with podofilox, an 85% solution of trichlo-
roacetic acid, cryocautery, or surgical excision. A self-treatment program utilizing 0.5% podofilox solution (Condylox) may be useful
for reliable patients and may prevent repetitive trips to the office.
Podofilox is applied to the wart twice a day for 3 days in row,
followed by 4 days of no treatment. This cycle can be repeated up
to 4 times and is safe and well-tolerated. Treatment will eradicate
the lesion but not the virus. Therefore patient education regarding
the chronic, often recurrent nature of HPV infection is critical. Colposcopy should be considered in all patients with external genital
condylomata, because cervical condylomata are difficult to see and
may lead to cervical cancer.

Hepatitis B Virus (HBV)

Primary care physicians may forget that HBV is a sexually transmitted disease. Heterosexuals with multiple partners have recently
replaced homosexual men as the highest risk group, accounting for
27% of new cases in 1990. Because HBV infection is preventable by
appropriate immunization, and because at least a third of cases
cannot be identified as "high-risk," new HBV immunization guidelines have been released. Current recommendations include giving
the first dose of hepatitis B vaccine in the newborn period, the
second dose at 1-2 months of age, and the third dose at 6-18 months
of age.

Genital Herpes Simplex Virus (HSV)

Herpes simplex virus (HSV) genital infections remain common
and problematic. Recurrence, large numbers of subclinical cases,
and lack of definitive cure complicate management. The classic
presentation with burning, itching, dysuria, extreme pain and tenderness of the vulva is hard to misdiagnose. If vesicular lesions are
present, rupturing a vesicle and rubbing the base of the ulcer with
a cotton-tipped swab for a culture is an easy diagnostic step. Oral
acyclovir (Zovirax) shortens the intensity and length of recurrent
and initial episodes.

Initial or recurrent HSV infection may be treated with acyclovir 200 milligrams orally 5 times per day for 5-7 days. Frequently recurring infections are treated continuously with acyclovir 800 milligrams once per day (or 400 milligrams twice daily) for 1 year. Patients with severe vulvar pain and/or urinary retention should be hospitalized and given acyclovir 5 milligrams per kilogram intravenously every 8 hours for 5 days or until symptoms are under control. Topical acyclovir has no role in treating genital HSV infection.

Pelvic Inflammatory Disease (PID)

PID is a generic term used to encompass infection of ovaries, tubes, uterus, and parametrium. It can be caused by a wide variety of aerobic and anaerobic bacteria, most commonly transmitted by sexual intercourse. PID is a diagnostic dilemma; an accurate bacteriological diagnosis is made in only about two thirds of cases. Minimal diagnostic criteria for the diagnosis of PID include lower abdominal tenderness, bilateral adnexal tenderness, and cervical motion tenderness. Compliant patients without evidence of sepsis or abscess can be treated as outpatients with close follow-up. Table 13.6 shows the current CDC recommendations for outpatient and inpatient treatment of PID. Posttreatment visits should include repeat cultures, pelvic examination, and counseling about STDs, fertility, and contraception.

Violence Against Women

Rape, "date-rape," domestic abuse, and sexual abuse of (usually) female children are problems that are extremely common, and also very difficult to detect and treat. Rural women may be especially vulnerable due to culture norms, poor socioeconomic status, lack of resources, isolation, and lack of safe refuge. The statistics, whether urban or rural, are dismal:

- One of every eight adult women has been raped.
- One of five visits to emergency rooms is related to domestic abuse.
- One of every four women in the United States has been beaten by a partner at least once.
- One of five girls (and 1 of 10 boys) has been sexually abused by the age of 18.

Table 13.6 Treatment of Pelvic Inflammatory Disease

OUTPATIENT THERAPY

Ceftriaxone 250 mg IM or Cefoxitin 2 g IM plus Probenecid 1 g po	PLUS	Doxycycline 100 mg po b.i.d. or Tetracycline 500 mg po q.i.d. for 10-14 days

For pregnant and allergic patients substitute
Erythromycin 500 mg po q.i.d. for 10-14 days

INPATIENT THERAPY

1. Doxycycline 100 mg po or IV b.i.d.	PLUS	Cefoxitin 2 g IV q 6 h or Cefotetan 2 g IV b.i.d.
2. Clindamycin 900 mg IV t.i.d.	PLUS	Gentamicin 2 mg/kg IV loading dose, then 1.5 mg/kg IV t.i.d. maintenance dose

Continue regimen 1 or 2 for 48 hours after clinical improvement, then switch to Doxycycline 100 mg po b.i.d. for 10-14 days.

Abused women may have multiple physical and psychiatric symptoms often seemingly unrelated to the abuse itself. The "simple" act of a pelvic examination by a male physician can be a terrifying reminder of the abuse event. Physicians need to be aware of the enormity of the problem and supportive to patients as they make decisions about their lives. The following guidelines will help:

- The victim must be assured of safety; no step should be taken without first ensuring the woman's safety. Shelters, relocation, and assurance of legal rights are equally important.
- Physicians must be supportive, nonjudgmental, and available.
- Marriage counseling is inappropriate and may be dangerous in an abusive relationship until the primary abuse situation is resolved.
- Physicians should know their local resources for shelters, counselors, hot lines, and patient education brochures. The National Domestic Violence Hotline number is 1-800-833-SAFE.

The Female Menopause

The population of postmenopausal women in the United States is increasing rapidly. Menopause and climacteric medicine are clinical challenges. Women are seeking answers to difficult questions. Because little research has been done on many of the areas of concern to menopausal women, dogmatic and rigid solutions are not appropriate. Individualization of treatment, information, and support will be necessary to help these women. A team approach involving nurses, dietitians, physical therapists, social workers, and psychologists may be effective and efficient.

The "hot flash" is usually the hallmark of the peri-menopause. It is a very vivid event, experienced by 80%-90% of peri-menopausal women, and it may begin 5 to 10 years before menopause. The hot flashes are more frequent and severe at night, and can lead to significant sleep disturbances. Estrogen, either orally or transdermally, is the most effective treatment. Initial control of symptoms can require greater doses of estrogen, which can be tapered with time. In those women who cannot take estrogen, progesterone and clonidine have been tried with some success.

Osteoporosis

This disease causes an absolute decrease in bone mass, thereby making bones susceptible to fracture with minimal trauma. Postmenopausal women are the most commonly affected, and loss of estrogen is a major contributing factor to a woman's risk of developing osteoporosis. Application of well-known risk factors (early menopause, under-average weight, small frame, cigarette smoking, alcohol abuse, sedentary lifestyle) can predict the disease in only about 50% of the population.

Prevention of osteoporosis should be viewed like a three-legged stool: exercise, adequate calcium intake, and estrogen replacement therapy. Weight-bearing exercises like walking, running, and aerobics will slow the rate of bone loss. However, total bone mass will still decrease, even in active, athletic women. Estrogen replacement therapy (ERT) prevents bone loss. The protective effect is maintained only while women continue on the replacement hormone. ERT has been shown to have a beneficial impact on bone mass even

in women over the age of 65, so there is no theoretical upper limit
for starting therapy. There appears to be no negative effect on bone
mass from the addition of progestational agents to ERT. Transder-
mal and oral estrogen are both effective in preventing osteoporosis.
ERT should be supplemented with a calcium intake of 1,000 milligrams per day.

New treatments and preventive agents for osteoporosis hold
some promise. Calcitonin is currently available only in injectable
form and is prohibitively expensive. Its role in preventing bone loss
and its analgesic properties make its use in acute vertebral compression fractures particularly appealing. The bisphosphonates (i.e., eti-
dronate) are currently being investigated and may also stabilize
bone mass. Long-term benefits and effects of these drugs are not
known.

Cardiovascular Disease

In the United States, cardiovascular disease (CVD) is the leading
cause of death for both women and men. ERT has been shown to
reduce the risk of CVD in postmenopausal women by 50%. Estrogen increases HDL cholesterol and lowers LDL-cholesterol. There
may also be a direct beneficial effect of estrogen on coronary arteries.

The use of a monthly progestin has clouded the beneficial picture
of ERT somewhat. Studies have not adequately assessed the effects
of progestin added to the various ERT regimens in current use. It
is likely that there is a dose-response relationship between pro-
gestins and their effects on lipoproteins. Therefore, choosing the
lowest progestational dose that protects the endometrium is probably wise.

Techniques of
Hormone Replacement Therapy (HRT)

Due to the potential cardiovascular and skeletal benefits, HRT
should be considered in most postmenopausal women, even if they
are not having symptoms of hormone deficiency. Absolute contraindications include a history of breast, cervical, uterine, or ovarian
cancer and recurrent thromboembolic disease. If a woman's uterus

is present, progestin is added sequentially or continuously to the estrogen. Because of the frequency of unwanted monthly withdrawal bleeding, a continuous regimen has been used: conjugated estrogen 0.625 milligram or micronized estradiol 1.0 milligram daily, plus medroxyprogesterone acetate 2.5 milligrams or norethindrone 0.35 milligram daily. After about 6 months of continuous HRT, bleeding usually ceases and the endometrium is atrophic. If the uterus is absent, estrogen alone may be used. The issue of the relation of ERT to breast cancer is controversial, but at this time it appears that any increase in risk, if present at all, is minimal.

Summary

Women's health has always been a major part of any rural family physician's practice. As new information from research becomes available about menopause, breast and cervical cancer, cardiovascular disease, and osteoporosis, physicians will have more to offer the women they regularly see.

Recommended Reading

Byyny, R. L., & Speroff, L. (1990). *A clinical guide for the care of older women*. Baltimore, MD: Williams & Wilkins.

Dickey, R. P. (1988). *Managing contraceptive pill patients*. Durant, OK: Creative Infomats.

Glass, R. (1988). *Office gynecology* (3rd ed.). Baltimore, MD: Williams & Wilkins.

Maderas, L., & Patterson, J. (1984). *Womancare*. New York: Avon.

Shepard, B. D., & Shepard, C. A. (1990). *The complete guide to women's health*. New York: Plume.

Speroff, L., Glass, R. M., & Kase, N. (1989). *Clinical gynecologic endocrinology and infertility*. Baltimore, MD: Williams & Wilkins.

Wilson, J. (1990). *Woman, your body, your health, the essential guide for well-being*. Orlando, FL: B.L.A. Publishing.

14

■ ■ ■

Caring for the AIDS Patient
in a Rural Practice

RICHARD D. SIMON, JR.

Introduction

Early in the AIDS epidemic most infected persons were treated in large tertiary care centers, but now persons with HIV infection and AIDS are being treated in most parts of the United States, including rural areas. This chapter focuses on the general principles of pathophysiology and transmission of the human immunodeficiency virus (HIV), early diagnosis and follow-up of HIV-infected patients, general principles of care of the patient with the severe immune deficiency characteristic of clinical acquired immunodeficiency syndrome (AIDS), end-of-life issues, and the role that rural health care workers should play as community educators.

HIV infection and its associated opportunistic infections are uncommon medical problems for most rural practitioners. Like other diseases with rapidly changing treatments, HIV infection and AIDS should not be managed by the rural physician alone. The physician will need support and the ability to consult with and refer to a physician or medical team with the clinical, social, and psychologic expertise necessary for the full spectrum of care for the AIDS patient. Regional or state educational conferences are good places for physicians to meet potential consultants and to find out about referral services. Identifying consultants before treating your first patient with AIDS is ideal.

Patients with advanced HIV infection and clinical AIDS require a multidisciplinary approach and experienced providers. The rural practitioner should develop open lines of communication with a secondary or tertiary care center familiar with the care of the AIDS patient.

Background

Since the initial 1981 AIDS reports, more than 200,000 cases of AIDS have been reported to the Centers for Disease Control and Prevention, and more than 140,000 persons have died of AIDS in the United States. AIDS has emerged as a leading cause of death among men and women under 45 years of age and of children 1 to 5 years of age in the United States. The most rapid rate of increase of new HIV infection is currently seen among adolescents and heterosexually active adults.

AIDS is a clinical syndrome characterized by declining immune function and increasing risk of opportunistic infections, unusual tumors, bone marrow suppression, neurologic disease, and general wasting that eventually results in death. AIDS is diagnosed when an individual with HIV infection develops one of several AIDS-defining opportunistic infections, tumors, or other clinical events. The progression from asymptomatic HIV infection to AIDS takes years.

Pathophysiology and Natural History

HIV binds to the CD4 marker present on the surfaces of certain cells, is internalized and uncoated, and its RNA is transcribed to DNA by viral reverse transcriptase. The DNA incorporates itself into the host's genome until it is activated, at which time the DNA is transcribed into new viral RNA and viral particles are produced. This process of replication usually results in the death of the host cell. Newly formed virus infects other CD4-positive cells, thus leading to the cycle of cell infection, viral replication and release, cell death, and spread of infection to other cells. This results in the gradual depletion of CD4-positive cells. Most CD4-positive cells are helper T-cell lymphocytes, whose function it is to coordinate a directed immune response.

Immune function declines in proportion to the decline in the CD4 T-cell count. A normal CD4 count ranges from about 600 to 1,200 cells per cubic milliliter, and HIV-infected patients usually have no symptoms or signs of immune suppression until the CD4 count drops below 500, when rather nonspecific symptoms of weight loss, low-grade fevers, and fatigue may occur. The incidence of opportunistic infections increases when the CD4 count drops below 200. Even with treatment the CD4 count continues to drop; death usually occurs when the CD4 count is less than 50.

Immediately after acute infection with HIV, blood virus levels are high. Partially protective antibodies form within 8 to 12 weeks of infection; 95% of HIV-infected individuals develop antibodies to HIV within 6 months. These antibodies may be responsible for the fall in blood virus levels and a slowing in the rate of fall of CD4 counts. After years of HIV-infection and declining CD4 levels severe immune dysfunction occurs; HIV antibody levels decline; HIV viremia increases; and eventually death occurs. Thus at the beginning and at the end of the natural history of HIV infection a person may have HIV infection but will test negative for antibodies to HIV.

Acute infection with HIV may manifest itself by a self-limited illness with fever, malaise, myalgias, headache, lymphadenopathy, pharyngitis, and skin rash lasting 1 to 3 weeks. This mononucleosis-like syndrome usually occurs a few weeks after acute infection with HIV. When it resolves, HIV infection remains clinically dormant and those infected remain asymptomatic, fully functional, healthy-appearing persons for years.

The clinical history of HIV infection can be classified as follows:

- Class I: acute infection
- Class II: asymptomatic infection (positive HIV antibody test but no symptoms)
- Class III: persistent generalized lymphadenopathy
- Class IV: AIDS

AIDS is defined as HIV infection and other opportunistic infections including Pneumocystis carinii, cytomegalovirus retinitis, Toxoplasma gondii, Histoplasma capsulatum, atypical mycobacterial infection, tumors such as Kaposi's sarcoma and central nervous system lymphoma, and neurologic disease.

Of infected individuals, 5% will develop clinical AIDS within 5 years of infection, 33% within 7 years of infection, and 50% within 10 years of infection. It is projected that 99% of infected individuals will develop AIDS within 16 years of infection and that eventually all will die of AIDS. A person infected with HIV will be completely asymptomatic for most of the duration of the infection; it is only during the last part of the natural history of HIV infection that symptoms and severe immune suppression occur. HIV infection should be viewed as a chronic illness rather than an acute illness. Many variables predict the progression from asymptomatic disease to AIDS but the most clinically useful is the CD4 count: 40% of HIV-infected individuals with a CD4 count less than 300 and 30% with a CD4 count between 300 and 399 will develop clinical AIDS within 3 years.

Transmission

The patterns of spread of HIV infection are predictable and have remained remarkably consistent since AIDS was first described. HIV infection is spread primarily by inoculation of blood by transfusion of blood or blood products, needle-sharing among intravenous drug abusers, needle stick exposure, infected blood on open wounds, and unsterile needle use; homosexual, bisexual, or heterosexual contact; and perinatal transmission.

The risk of transmission of infection is related to the inoculum of infectious virus as well as to the location of the exposure. Because viremia is highest early in HIV infection and again late in HIV infection, HIV-infected persons are probably more infectious either very early or very late in the course of the disease. The risk of HIV infection to a patient receiving a transfusion of HIV-infected blood is 90%. Of women who routinely have unprotected intercourse with HIV-infected partners, 80% will develop HIV infection over a period of 18 months, whereas only 18% of women routinely using condoms during intercourse with HIV-infected partners will develop HIV infection over the same time. Thirty percent of babies born to HIV-infected mothers will develop HIV infection. The risk of deep scalpel cut transmission from an HIV-infected patient to a health care worker is approximately 17% per exposure, and the risk of needle stick transmission is only 0.3%-0.4% per exposure. There is a high efficiency of HIV transmission with a large inoculum of infected blood as occurs in transfusion, a very low efficiency of transmission through percutaneous exposure, and no risk from casual nonsexual exposure.

Ninety-nine percent of HIV-positive health care workers become infected through the usual sexual and intravenous routes of transmission. The prevalence of HIV among health care workers is not significantly different from that of the general population, implying that caring for HIV-infected patients does not constitute a risk for HIV infection. By using universal precautions (Table 14.1) the small risk to health care workers can be reduced even further. All medical personnel must be instructed in the principles of universal precautions.

More than 60% of AIDS cases reported in the United States are contracted through sexual activity. The fraction of cases attributable to homosexual and bisexual activity has decreased by 8%, and the fraction due to heterosexual activity has increased by 40% in the last 3 years. Few heterosexually active persons view themselves as being at risk for HIV infection, and they need to be reminded of this risk.

Approximately 25% of AIDS cases in the United States are linked to intravenous drug use. Infection may be the result of needle sharing or increased sexual activity associated with certain types of drug use, especially cocaine use. Blood transfusions account for 2% of HIV infection, 1.6% is due to perinatal transmission, and 6% of cases have no identifiable source, although most of these have not yet been fully investigated.

Testing

Serologic tests detect evidence of HIV infection before symptoms occur. The enzyme-linked immunosorbent assay (ELISA) and Western blot tests measure the presence of antibody to HIV; these tests do not test for the virus itself, although such tests are available in research settings and may soon be available for general use. The ELISA test is used only as a screening test because of the low number of false negative results and the high number of false positive results. In screening with the ELISA test, few infected individuals are missed; but a more specific test (the Western blot test) is needed to separate true positives from false positives. Patients should not be told of positive ELISA results until they are confirmed by Western blot testing in a reference laboratory.

Because of the serious nature and consequences, HIV test results should not be given over the phone. A return visit should be scheduled for all patients having an HIV test. At the follow-up visit of a

Table 14.1 Universal Precautions for All Health Care Workers

HAND WASHING

Before and after each patient contact or contact with potentially infective material.

GLOVES

Wear gloves if likely to come into contact with blood, secretions, excretions, body fluids, or tissues. Double glove during invasive surgical procedures. Health care workers with open skin lesions should refrain from patient care activities.

GOWNS

Wear when clothing is likely to be soiled.

MASKS AND EYE PROTECTION

Wear when splashes are likely to occur.

NEEDLE STICK PRECAUTIONS

Puncture-resistant containers should be available in all areas where "sharps" are to be used. Needles should not be resheathed or otherwise manipulated and they should never be placed on beds, furniture, or waste cans. If resheathing is necessary, a single-handed technique should be used. Never walk across a room with an exposed "sharp." The vast majority of needle stick exposures can be prevented!

LAUNDRY

Standard hospital procedures are satisfactory.

WASTE DISPOSAL

Place in waterproof bags and dispose of in accordance with local rules. Decontaminate items saturated with body fluids.

STERILIZATION AND DISINFECTION

Clean instruments, decontaminate (soak in germicidal solution), then sterilize.

ENVIRONMENTAL CONTAMINATION

Wash surface with disinfectant that is viricidal and mycobactericidal; a 1:10 dilution of sodium hypochlorite (household bleach) is satisfactory. Have workers cleaning such spills use universal precautions!

Table 14.2 HIV Risk Assessment

Are you sexually active?
How many sexual partners have you had in the past 10 years?
How many sexual partners do you currently have?
Do you use condoms? How often?
Have any of your partners ever tested positive for HIV?
Have any of your partners ever had AIDS?
Have you been treated for a sexually transmitted disease (gonorrhea, pelvic inflammatory disease, chlamydia, syphilis, venereal warts) in the past 10 years?
Do you use recreational drugs? Do you use or share needles?
Have you had any blood transfusions between 1978 and 1986 (inquire about surgeries and accidents)?
Are you interested in being tested for HIV?

patient with a negative HIV test, the result should be given to the patient and educational materials should be briefly reviewed. In particular, the limitations of the HIV antibody test must be reviewed. Except in very unusual cases, an HIV test should not be done without the patient's permission. Legislation on this issue varies from state to state.

Counseling and Diagnosis

The vast majority of the care required for HIV-infected persons is well within the domain of primary care and not unlike other chronic illness such as diabetes, heart failure, ischemic heart disease, hypertension, and chronic lung disease. Because early diagnosis leads to early treatment, prolonged survival, and decreased spread of infection, an HIV risk assessment should be part of every routine exam (Table 14.2).

Routine exams such as school exams, sports physicals, insurance exams, driver's exams, and periodic physical exams provide the opportunity for the practitioner to assess HIV risks and to educate patients about HIV disease. The history and education should be done in a nonjudgmental, nonprejudicial manner. Topics that need to be covered include the viral nature of HIV infection, the prolonged asymptomatic phase of HIV infection, the clinical syndrome AIDS, the methods of transmission of HIV, the concepts of safer sex

Table 14.3 Safe Sex Guidelines

SAFEST (NO RISK)

> Abstention from sexual contact
> Monogamous relationship between two uninfected persons
> Self-masturbation
> Touching, petting, holding hands, hugging

SAFER (RISK PROBABLY ZERO)

> Partner masturbation (if no cuts on hand or if condom used)
> Dry kissing

LOW RISK (BUT NOT ZERO RISK)

> Vaginal sex with proper use of intact, new condom
> Wet kissing
> Fellatio with proper use of intact, new condom

PROBABLY SOME RISK

> Fellatio without use of condom
> Cunnilingus (risk probably higher during menstrual flow and if there
>   are sores on the mouth)
> Receptive anal intercourse with proper use of intact, new condom

HIGH RISK

> Unprotected vaginal intercourse with an infected partner
> Unprotected receptive anal intercourse with an infected partner
> Numerous partners

(Table 14.3), treatment of HIV infection, and the limitations of the HIV antibody test. This needs to be done periodically with all patients because some patients will not feel free to discuss their sexual activities or drug use.

Patients with a history of high-risk behaviors should be offered HIV testing. It is also recommended that patients being treated for sexually transmitted diseases be offered HIV testing. Because of the recent association of tuberculosis (TB) and HIV, patients with recently diagnosed TB or a positive PPD should be offered HIV testing. It is important to tell patients that they can be tested anonymously at public health offices and HIV centers if they would prefer.

Table 14.4 Laboratory Studies for HIV Infected Patients

INITIAL LABORATORY STUDIES

CBC, ESR, chemistry profile, chest X ray, urinalysis, CD4 count, cytomegalovirus antibodies, Hepatitis B surface antigen and antibody,
Toxoplasmosis antibody titers, PPD, VDRL, Pap test for women.

YEARLY LABORATORY STUDIES

VDRL, PPD, Pap test for women. Other studies are ordered based on
clinical needs. CD4 count depending on the clinical status (see text).

The Patient With a Positive
HIV Test

If the confirmatory Western blot is positive, at least 30 minutes
should be scheduled for the follow-up appointment. A positive
Western blot is devastating news and must be presented honestly
and compassionately. It is important to pay careful attention to the
patient's reaction and emotional state. Occasionally depression or
suicidal ideation may necessitate hospitalization. The health care
provider's greatest contribution to the patient's well-being at this
stage is support.

The patient with newly diagnosed HIV infection faces enormous
psychological and social problems. He must decide with whom he
is going to share this news. He faces the possibility of losing his job,
friends, intimate relationships, and family support, and of course
must face his own mortality. Letting the patient know that you will
not abandon him, that support groups are available, and that there
is a plan of care is critical. The primary care practitioner must also
assure the patient that medical confidentiality will be maintained.

During the second visit, a complete history and physical exam
should done, if it has not previously been performed. An immunization history should be obtained and baseline laboratory studies
should be obtained (Table 14.4). The patient may wish to bring his
or her sexual partner, family, or significant other to this visit. Sufficient time should be allowed to answer questions and to address
concerns that all the parties may have. Regional support services

Table 14.5 Recommended Immunizations for HIV-Infected Persons

DIPHTHERIA AND TETANUS TOXOIDS

Two doses intramuscularly 1 month apart; third dose 6 months later. Booster every 10 years.

MEASLES, MUMPS, RUBELLA

If born after 1956 or lacking in protective antibodies. Appears safe even in symptomatic disease but consultation with tertiary care center suggested if CD4 < 200 as there is debate about this. One dose subcutaneously, repeated 1 month later.

HEPATITIS B VACCINE

Give if seronegative. Two doses intramuscularly 1 month apart with third dose at 6 months. Check titers.

INFLUENZA

Given yearly just before the anticipated flu season.

PNEUMOCOCCAL VACCINE

Given once with booster in 6 years.

HEMOPHILUS INFLUENZAE TYPE B CONJUGATE VACCINE

Dosing schedule is not defined in adults but recommended for HIV-infected patients.

ENHANCED POTENCY INACTIVATED POLIOVIRUS VACCINE

Two doses subcutaneously 1 month apart with third dose at 6 months. Avoid the live oral poliovirus vaccine.

should be offered again. Another visit should be scheduled to review the laboratory studies.

During the third visit laboratory results are explained and the plans for monitoring and treating the HIV infection are developed and reviewed. Appropriate immunizations should be offered (Table 14.5), and follow-up is scheduled.

HIV Infection and Moderate
Immunosuppression (CD4 = 200-500)

Once the CD4 count drops to less than 500, symptoms of low-grade fever, weight loss, generalized fatigue, lymphadenopathy, and diarrhea may occur. Most opportunistic infections do not occur with a CD4 count greater than 200. Early use of zidovudine (AZT) delays the development of AIDS in asymptomatic HIV-infected patients with CD4 counts of less than 500. Even if the drug is not instituted until after clinical AIDS develops, zidovudine offers survival advantage. In addition to zidovudine, dideoxyinosine (DDI) and zalcitabine (DDC) are currently approved by the Food and Drug Administration for treatment of HIV infections.

AZT should be given in a dose of 200 milligrams three times daily when the CD4 count falls below 500. Adverse effects include nausea, vomiting, fatigue, headache, confusion, anemia, and neutropenia. A complete blood count should be checked periodically to monitor hematologic toxicity. In the presence of anemia and a low serum erythropoietin level, erythropoietin administration may elevate the hemoglobin so that AZT can be continued.

At this stage of infection, common pathogens generally will be found during bouts of acute illness. Two common pathogens that are particularly worrisome are tuberculosis and syphilis.

Tuberculosis tends to occur in the HIV-infected patient when immunity is only moderately suppressed (average CD4 count 300-400). A yearly purified protein derivative test (PPD) is recommended for all HIV-infected patients. An HIV-infected patient presenting with a cough should have three early morning sputum collections for acid fast stain, culture, and sensitivity. Delayed diagnosis of TB in the HIV-infected patient is associated with premature death. Failure to obtain three morning sputum collections for acid fast stain and culture is the most common reason for delayed diagnosis.

Isoniazid (INH) 300 milligrams per day for 1 year should be offered to any patient with a PPD induration of 5 mm or more. If clinical TB occurs, treatment should be initiated with INH 300 milligrams, rifampin 600 milligrams, and pyrazinamide 15-25 milligrams per kilogram given daily for at least 2 months. Ethambutol 15-25 milligrams per kilogram daily should be added if there is the possibility of INH-resistant organisms. After 2 months of 3- or 4-drug therapy, INH and rifampin should be continued for an additional 9 months, or at least 6 months after cultures have become negative. Therapy may be modified based on sensitivity results.

Primary syphilis involves the central nervous system (CNS) most of the time, even in immunocompetent hosts. The usual dose of penicillin for syphilis (2.4 million units intramuscularly) does not penetrate the CNS in levels necessary to eradicate CNS sanctuary sites. However, the immunocompetent host is able to eradicate the presumably small numbers of spirochetes remaining in the CNS. The HIV-infected host is unable to mount a sufficient immune response to eradicate CNS sanctuary sites of syphilis and thus may not respond as completely to treatment. Any HIV-infected patient with a positive VDRL must have a cerebrospinal fluid (CSF) VDRL performed.

In a patient with a positive serum VDRL and a negative CSF VDRL, primary therapy consists of either benzathine penicillin 2.4 million units intramuscularly every week for 3 weeks; procaine penicillin 1.2 million units intramuscularly and probenecid 500 milligrams orally daily for 14 days; or ceftriaxone 1 gram intramuscularly daily or every other day for 10 to 14 days for penicillin-allergic patients. The effectiveness of doxycycline has not been well studied in HIV infected patients.

If the CSF VDRL is positive, aqueous penicillin G 12 million units intravenously and probenecid 500 milligrams orally is given each day for 10 days, followed by benzathine penicillin 2.4 million units intramuscularly each week for 3 weeks. The serum and CSF VDRL are repeated at 3- to 6-month intervals. If positivity remains or recurs, the patient is retreated.

Kaposi's sarcoma (KS) may occur in the HIV-infected patient with relatively high CD4 counts. Any suspicious pigmented cutaneous lesion in an HIV-infected patient should be biopsied. In advanced AIDS, pulmonary KS may occur and has a poor prognosis, even with aggressive chemotherapy. Because there are no fixed protocols for the management of KS, tertiary care center consultation is highly recommended.

HIV Infection and Severe Immunosuppression (CD4 < 200)

A CD4 count of less than 200 signifies the presence of severe immune dysfunction. There is debate about whether CD4 monitoring is useful once it has fallen to less than 200. Should a sudden rapid drop in the CD4 count occur, or should the CD4 count drop to less than 50, one could argue that resistance to zidovudine has occurred and DDI or DDC should be added. The area of retroviral drug therapy is rapidly changing and telephone consultation with a tertiary care center is recommended.

Prophylaxis against Pneumocystis carinii should be started when the CD4 count falls to less than 200. One double-strength tablet of trimethoprim-sulfamethoxazole daily is recommended; this may also afford some protection against Hemophilus influenzae and Toxoplasma gondii. Side effects such as fever, rash, bone marrow suppression, and abnormal liver function tests are common. Other prophylactic regimens include dapsone 25 to 50 milligrams daily or 100 milligrams twice weekly, or aerosolized pentamidine at 300 milligrams per month. Pentamidine is convenient but quite expensive and has been associated with extra-pulmonary Pneumocystis infection.

Because serious fungal infections are quite common when the CD4 count is less than 50, it is reasonable to add prophylactic fluconazole at a dose 200 milligrams per day. Fluconazole is well tolerated, it penetrates the central nervous system well, and efficacy in maintenance therapy has been demonstrated in AIDS patients with a variety of systemic fungal infections. Fluconazole is not approved by the FDA for prophylactic purposes.

Clinical AIDS

Multiple opportunistic infections characterize the end stage of HIV infection and are the direct result of progressive immune dysfunction. Because of the severe immune deficiency state that occurs in AIDS, the patient with AIDS is not able to mount an effective immune response to acute infections. This greatly alters the presentation of infections with both pathogenic and opportunistic organisms. Clinical presentations are often nonspecific and often overlap with symptoms of HIV infection itself. Common infections still occur, and can present in unusual ways. Appropriate laboratory specimens are crucial for proper diagnosis.

Once the type of infection is identified by culture, biopsy, or serology, appropriate antibiotic therapy is indicated. Emphasis should also be placed on symptomatic support and care. In immunocompetent hosts, antibiotic therapy for infection provides a degree of protection by decreasing the infectious load so that the host's immune system can better handle the infection. Because there is little immune response in the AIDS patient, infections should be treated with high dose initial remission induction therapy followed by lower dose chronic maintenance therapy, often for the remainder of the patient's life.

Patients with AIDS commonly have several coexisting infections that may be simultaneously diagnosed or that may occur over the course of time. It is common for patients with AIDS to be on several different antibiotics at the same time.

In the ill person with a CD4 count less than 200, blood, sputum, cerebrospinal fluid, and urine should be cultured for routine organisms, mycobacteria, fungus, and virus. Buffy coat blood culture for virus is particularly useful in the diagnosis of cytomegalovirus infection. Serologic tests are often quite helpful in the diagnoses of cryptococcosis, histoplasmosis, coccidioidomycosis, and toxoplasmosis. Culturing biopsied tissue for routine organisms, mycobacteria, fungus, and virus can also be very helpful. Microscopic examination of early morning sputum by experienced laboratory personnel may reveal Pneumocystis carinii or mycobacterial infections. Examination of stools for ova and parasites, including Cryptosporidia, is frequently helpful. Although most rural hospitals and labs cannot perform all of these functions, arrangements can be made to transfer specimens and fluids to an appropriate reference laboratory.

The complexity of the patient with the severe immunosuppression characteristic of clinical AIDS requires a multidisciplinary approach that is difficult in the rural community where resources are limited. Timely telephone consultations can help the rural physician know what laboratory tests to order, what therapeutic approaches to consider, and when to transfer the patient to the tertiary care center.

The patient with AIDS often takes numerous medications, many of which require intravenous dosing. Most can be managed at home with the help of home health nurses and frequent house calls. Symptomatic treatment is very important as is support from a tertiary care team.

End-of-Life Issues

The basic problem in HIV infection is progressive and relentless immune dysfunction. At some point during their illnesses most HIV-infected patients realize that further aggressive, curative care is no longer helpful to them. At this stage the purpose of medicine properly shifts from that of restoring health and life to that of providing for comfort. Treatment should focus on providing the dying person with AIDS with a kind and gentle death, avoiding needless painful diagnostic and therapeutic procedures, controlling diarrhea as much as possible, and providing pain relief with narcotic analgesics without fear of addiction. At this stage a hospice approach can be very helpful.

A hospital bed, a bedside commode, a wheelchair, and oxygen can be delivered to the patient's home if needed. Analgesics such as morphine sulfate should be administered liberally to relieve discomfort. Tricyclic antidepressants, often in fairly low doses, can be very helpful in pain control. The use of patient-controlled subcutaneous delivery systems of analgesics is very effective and well received. When death is inevitable, many patients prefer to die in the comfort and familiarity of their homes with their loved ones present.

Doctor (*Docere*—To Teach)

In addition to caring for the individual patient with HIV infection, health care practitioners have a professional obligation to educate their communities about HIV infection. Because the methods of transmission are well known and potentially within an individual's control, the rate of spread of HIV can be decreased if appropriate measures are taken. The rural physician who publicly speaks about HIV infection and who is willing to care for HIV-infected individuals sends a very strong message to his or her community: that HIV infection is a disease like any other disease; it is not a curse or a punishment from God. Although AIDS is an infectious disease, it is not a very contagious disease. A person who does not engage in high-risk behaviors has virtually no risk of contracting HIV infection. Rural physicians can help the community, businesses, and schools deal with HIV-infected persons in a rational, compassionate, and humane manner.

How to Keep Up to Date

It is understandable that many rural physicians feel they are ill prepared to care for HIV infected patients. Such practitioners need not feel alone; all health care workers caring for HIV-infected persons feel ill prepared. This is a new illness, and treatment strategies are not yet satisfactory and are changing rapidly. Several readily accessible sources of information about AIDS are available (see the Resources).

The practitioner who wishes to learn most efficiently should consider attending AIDS courses held periodically in most metropolitan areas. These courses lead the novice as well as the experienced practitioner through the natural history, treatment strategies, and social implications of HIV infection.

AIDS Clinical Care is a superb monthly periodical with the purpose of helping the practitioner care for patients with HIV disease. It is easily read, not highly technical, and brief. For the physician who wishes more in-depth knowledge, appropriate references are provided. Each issue is generally devoted to one or two major topics. A special section devoted to primary care of the HIV-infected person has recently been added; and there is a question and answer section that often is a source of "pearls" of clinical wisdom not found in textbooks.

The AIDS Knowledge Base: A Textbook on HIV Disease From the University of California, San Francisco and the San Francisco General Hospital is a very complete, well-indexed, useful reference. This is available in textbook form and through computer modem telephone connections. The on-line version is updated frequently.

The most effective way to learn about HIV disease, however, is to care for patients with HIV disease. At first, frequent telephone consultation with a regional tertiary care center specializing in AIDS will be required, but with time the frequency of telephone consultation will decrease. HIV-infected patients and their families will be grateful for the care they receive and they will be especially appreciative that they can be cared for in their local communities. The

206 EXPLORING RURAL MEDICINE

intangible rewards for caring for such patients and for helping one's community deal with this illness are enormous.

Recommended Reading

Abramowicz, A. (Ed.). (1991). Drugs for AIDS and Associated Infections. *Medical Letter on Drugs and Therapeutics, 33,* 95-102.

Centers for Disease Control. (1981). Pneumocystis pneumonia—Los Angeles. *Morbidity & Mortality Weekly Review, 30,* 250-252.

Centers for Disease Control. (1991). The HIV/AIDS Epidemic: The First 10 Years. *Morbidity & Mortality Weekly Review, 40,* 357-369.

Fauci, A. S. (Moderator). (1991). Immunopathogenic mechanisms in human immunodeficiency virus (HIV) infection. *Annals of Internal Medicine, 114,* 678-693.

Greene, W. C. (1991). The molecular biology of human immunodeficiency virus Type 1 infection. *New England Journal of Medicine, 324,* 308-317.

Moore, R. D., Hidalgo, J., Sugland, B. W., & Chaisson, R. E. (1991). Zidovudine and the natural history of the acquired immunodeficiency syndrome. *New England Journal of Medicine, 324,* 1412-1416.

Sloan, E. M., Pitt, E., Chiarello, R. J., & Nemo, G. J. (1991). HIV testing: State of the art. *Journal of the American Medical Association, 266,* 2861-2866.

Veenstra, R. J., & Gluck, J. C. (1991). Access to information about AIDS. *Annals of Internal Medicine, 114,* 320-324.

Yarchoan, R., Venzon, D. J., Pluda, J. M., et al. (1991). CD4 count and the risk of death in patients infected with HIV receiving antiretroviral therapy. *Annals of Internal Medicine, 115,* 184-189.

Resources

Sources of Information About AIDS

"The Clinical Care of the AIDS Patient."
Postgraduate Programs, Department of Medicine
521 Parnassus, Room C-405
University of California-San Francisco
Box 0656
San Francisco, CA 94143-0656
(415) 896-0486

AIDS Clearing House
(800) 458-5231

AIDS Clinical Care.
The Massachusetts Medical Society
P.O. Box 9085
Waltham, MA 02254-9085
(800) 843-6356

Hecht, F. M., & Soloway, B. (Eds.). (1990). *HIV infection: A primary care approach.* Waltham: Massachusetts Medical Society.

The AIDS Knowledge Base: A Textbook on HIV Disease From the University of California, San Francisco and the San Francisco General Hospital (Philip T. Cohen et al., eds.).

Available from the Massachusetts Medical Society. Also available via computer modem through:

BRS Information Technologies
8000 Westpark Drive
McLean, VA 22102
(800) 289-4277

15
■ ■ ■

Treatment of Patients
With Terminal Cancer

WAYNE H. THALHUBER

Introduction

Physicians are faced with a vast array of evolving health care issues. Nowhere is change more apparent than in the right-to-die movement. In 1991 the U.S. Congress passed the Patient Self Determination Act requiring hospitals to provide information concerning living wills and to inquire about their existence for each patient. Family autonomy allows families the right to decide life and death issues for incapacitated patients without outside interference.

Most of the focus has been on life-extending technology and on life-ending procedures such as euthanasia and assisted suicide. As society looks at the costs and benefits of health care, however, the concept of futile care has emerged.

Futility in medical care is defined as treatment that simply does not work. A futile treatment has an extremely low efficacy, and a physician has no obligation to offer a treatment that is not expected to be effective. Initially applied to cardiopulmonary resuscitation in nursing home patients who are chronically ill or demented, futility has been extended to cancer therapy.

This chapter deals with the recognition and follow-up of patients in whom further cancer treatment may be futile. A classification of therapeutic benefit in cancer patients is proposed and illustrated. This is especially relevant to rural physicians who must help patients determine the value of further therapy after the surgeon or oncologist in the tertiary care center completes primary or secondary treatment. The rural primary care physician is the advisor whose opinion the family is most likely to seek.

What Care Is Futile?

Patients with metastatic or recurrent cancer can be grouped according to their anticipated response to subsequent therapy into three categories:

1. Therapeutic Benefit Marginal (TBM)
2. Therapeutic Benefit Unlikely (TBU)
3. Therapeutic Benefit Futile (TBF)

Therapeutic Benefit Marginal

TBM defines a group of patients with metastatic cancer whose response rate to any known treatment is approximately 20%. These patients have metastases at the time of initial treatment or develop metastases early after initial therapy. Radiation or chemotherapy in this group usually controls the disease process and allows for continued quality of life for a time, but cure is not anticipated.

Plan of Care for TBM Patients

1. Inform the patient and the family of the extent of the disease.
2. Describe the available treatment options, including expected response rate and side effects.
3. Present chemotherapy as a 3- to 6-month trial with an explanation of how remission status will be reassessed.
4. If therapy fails, inform the patient and offer second opinions and access to any experimental protocols.
5. Open "do not resuscitate" discussion with patient and family.
6. Discuss living wills.
7. Openly discuss and discourage quackery.
8. Confront the fear of abandonment and discuss hospices, including pain management and end-of-life issues.

Therapeutic Benefit Unlikely

The TBU group of patients has failed primary therapy. Additional therapeutic interventions have a low probability of remission induction (7% to 20%). This group of patients includes the elderly who are unable to tolerate side effects of treatment and those with other chronic disease processes that preclude therapy.

Plan of Care for TBU Patients

1. A family care conference is a very productive method of informing the patient and family of the advanced stage and progression of the disease.
2. Discuss the unlikely benefits of available second- and third-line therapies. Help the family understand the risk/benefit ratio of further treatment.
3. Inform patients of the availability of any experimental protocols.
4. Open discussion of "do not resuscitate" and likely length-of-life issues.
5. Strongly encourage participation in a hospice program.
6. Confront issues of pain management and abandonment.
7. Offer help as an advocate for the patient and family.

Therapeutic Benefit Futile

TBF describes a group of patients with metastatic disease who have either failed primary therapy or who are not candidates for primary therapy and in whom subsequent treatment has a low probability (less than 7%) of remission or of maintaining survival.

A distinction must be made between a treatment's effect and its benefit. A given treatment may affect some portion of the patient such as a decreased tumor size but not benefit the patient as a whole, neither prolonging life nor improving its quality. Treatment that fails to be beneficial even though it may have a localized effect is futile.

Plan of Care for TBF Patients

1. Warn the patient and family about the "chemotherapy to casket" syndrome. Inform them that further therapy is futile.

2. Discuss anticipated progression and effects of the disease.
3. Define palliative care and emphasize the importance of pain control and emotional and physical support.
4. Strongly encourage participation in a hospice program. Introduce the family to a hospice representative.
5. Expand treatment to include the needs of the other family members.

Assessing Futility of Treatment

Determining the likely success of further therapy in any patient is difficult. Whenever possible it is important to consult an oncologist who can assess the patient and the potential effect of established and experimental treatment regimens. However, it is useful for the primary care physician to have a general knowledge of the efficacy of treatment in common types of cancer.

The following is a review of common cancers and current therapies based on information in *Clinical Oncology,* published by the American Cancer Society in 1991. Because oncology treatment changes rapidly, this should be considered only as a guideline, and updated information should obtained from the most current sources.

Non-Small Cell Lung Cancer
(NSCLC)

This cancer is the leading cause of cancer deaths in men, and the incidence is rapidly increasing in women: 75% of all patients have unresectable disease at diagnosis. Radiation therapy for localized inoperable disease results in survival rates of only 15% at 2 years and 5% at 5 years. The addition of daily cisplatin improves the 2-year survival rate to 26% and the 3-year rate to 16%.

In patients with metastatic NSCLC, a trial of four different chemotherapy regimens resulted in no better than 18% one-year survival. Surviving patients were those less than 60 years of age and with no liver or bone metastases. Toxicity was often severe, with 40% of patients developing life-threatening or lethal leukopenia. Severe vomiting, renal toxicity, and neurological complications were also frequently encountered.

Using the proposed futility classification, we would place patients with locally inoperable NSCLC in the TBM category. Those with metastatic disease fall into the TBU group, with rapid conversion into the TBF if no response to treatment is seen in 3 to 6 months or if toxicity develops. Those over 60 years of age with metastatic disease fall into the TBF group at the time of diagnosis.

Breast Cancer

Localized breast cancer should be considered potentially curable in all women. Metastatic breast cancer is generally incurable despite hormonal and chemotherapeutic efforts. Objective response of metastatic breast cancer to combination chemotherapy occurs in 40%-70% of women with a median survival of 18 months. Salvage regimens following failure of initial therapy are used but responses are poor and of short duration.

Hormonal treatment in women with metastatic disease and tumor estrogen or progesterone receptors frequently produces good initial results with few side effects. However, most patients eventually become resistant to treatment.

Following failure of initial chemotherapy or of second-line hormonal therapy, these women will be in the TBU category. As the disease progresses to include visceral or central nervous system involvement and treatment is not improving quality of life, the patients will fall into the TBF category.

Colon Cancer

Metastatic colon cancer (Duke's D) has a 5-year survival rate of 5% or less with the most effective form of therapy. The addition of leucovorin (folinic acid) to 5-fluorouracil does improve the response rate to 15% or 20% but has not increased the survival rate. Therefore, Duke's D colon neoplasms would be classified in the TBU group, advancing to the TBF group as initial response fails.

Prostate Cancer

Metastatic prostate cancer is best treated by hormonal therapy, estrogen, or orchiectomy. Cure is unusual, with median survival in ambulatory patients without other serious illness of 2 to 3 years. Leuprolide alone is equivalent to orchiectomy; when the antiandrogen flutamide is added, improved survival is seen in patients with minimal disease.

When metastatic prostate cancer becomes resistant to hormonal manipulation there is no further effective chemotherapy. Radiation treatment may be useful for symptom relief but any chemotherapy should be considered in the category TBF.

Renal Cell Cancer

There is no effective chemotherapy or hormonal therapy for metastatic renal cell carcinoma, and so this cancer would be considered TBF. Newer treatments are currently under investigation and may be available under an experimental protocol.

The use of interferon-alpha has resulted in response rates of 10% to 20%. Combining interleukin-2 and lymphokine-activated killer cells has generated some early enthusiasm because some complete remissions have resulted. This emphasizes the need to update information with the latest data available. A cancer in the TBF category at diagnosis may be reclassified TBU or even TBM with the introduction of new treatment modalities.

Leukemia

Acute nonlymphocytic leukemia usually goes into remission following intensive chemotherapy. The use of consolidated or maintenance chemotherapy offers complete remission in only 25% of patients. This would place initial treatment in the TBM category. Following relapse, additional treatment to reinduce remission is successful in less than 20% of patients; 5-year survival is less than 5%. Therapy in this situation would be considered TBF.

However, allogenic bone marrow transplantation during relapse in young patients with perfect HLA/MLC matches does have a 45% to 65% chance of 2- to 5-year disease-free remissions. Treatment following relapse after marrow transplantation is unlikely to be effective and is classified as TBF.

Chronic myelogenous leukemia (CML) in the chronic phase is treated to control the white count and symptoms. This treatment is considered TBM. Once a blastic crisis has occurred, the remission rate with the most aggressive treatment is only 20%; short-term survival is the only practical goal. Chemotherapy would be considered TBU and rapidly slipping to TBF.

Allogenic bone marrow transplant offers a potential cure for CML and is usually done early in the chronic phase in patients less than 40 years of age. Long-term disease-free survival for this subgroup approaches 50%.

Pancreatic Cancer

Carcinoma of the pancreas has a dismal prognosis. If not resectable, the survival rate is 20% for 1 year and 3% for 5 years. Metastatic pancreatic carcinoma is designated as TBU, rapidly slipping to TBF.

Ovarian Cancer

Of women found to have ovarian cancer, 75% present with Stage III or IV disease. Cyclophosphamide and cisplatin produce response rates of 40% in this group. For women who respond to six cycles of chemotherapy, a second-look operation is recommended to remove residual disease and instill intraperitoneal chemotherapy if indicated.

Taxol is a promising new agent used for salvage therapy for recurrent disease, but only a few patients have received this drug. Once metastatic disease has been shown to be resistant to taxol, additional therapy would be considered TBF. However, it was not long ago that initial therapy would have been considered TBF.

Summary

This chapter has developed a framework to help family physicians and general internists care for their patients with metastatic cancer. Although family physicians may not order the chemotherapy, it is often the primary care physician to whom the family turns for advice about further therapeutic attempts.

Physicians may be slow to realize that the clinical decline of their patients implies the futility of further care. The therapeutic response classification described in this chapter enables the physician to emphasize the positive aspects of terminal care and to recognize the relative ineffectiveness of additional therapy. The proposed classification offers physicians a positive framework for openly discussing metastatic disease processes at a time difficult for both patient and physician.

Recommended Reading

Blackhall, L. J. (1987). Must we always use CPR? *New England Journal of Medicine, 317*, 1281-1285.

Lantos, J. D., Singer, P. A., Walker, R. M., et al. (1989). The illusion of futility in clinical practice. *American Journal of Medicine, 87*, 81-84.

Holleb, A. I., Fine, D. J., & Murray, G. P. (Eds.). (1991). *Clinical oncology.* Atlanta, GA: American Cancer Society.

Murphy, D. J. (1988). Do not resuscitate orders: Time for reappraisal. *Journal of the American Medical Association, 260*, 2098-2101.

Schiedermayer, D. L. (1988). The decision to forgo CPR in the elderly. *Journal of the American Medical Association, 260*, 2096-2097.

Schneiderman, L. J., Jecker, N. S., & Jonsen, A. R. (1990). Medical futility: Its meaning and ethical implications. *Annals of Internal Medicine, 112*, 949-954.

Youngner, S. J. (1988). Who defines futility? *Journal of the American Medical Association, 260*, 2094-2095.

16

■ ■ ■

Caring for Dying Patients and Their Families

PATRICIA M. COLE

NORMA WYLIE

You matter because you are you. You matter to the last moment of your life, and we will do all we can not only to help you die peacefully, but also to live until you die.

—Dame Cicely Saunders

Orchestrating care for dying patients is one of the most challenging and potentially one of the most satisfying aspects of rural practice. The personal physician is essential to a successful collaboration between patient, family, and health care system. Seldom does medical education provide guidelines for this universal process. Dying patients evoke in us uncomfortable emotions: Anger at our inability to cure, uncertainty about our role, denial that we have feelings at all, fear as we face our own deaths. Dying patients exhaust us and shake our comfortable professional demeanor. American culture avoids the issue of death, even as we spend huge amounts of money on terminally ill patients.

"Good death" occurs best when the dying patient is alert, relatively free from painful symptoms, and supported by family and a compassionate and competent medical care team. The doctor and team ought to model empathetic, clear communication with patients and help family members do the same. Usually patient and family can reconcile, finish old business, find spiritual support, and make well-informed end-of-life decisions, if adequately informed and helped to manage symptoms. Nursing care, intensive treatments, and much education will be done by others, but the patient's personal physician should understand enough to manage the process. The purpose of this chapter is to review current concepts on hospice, right of self-determination legislation, and pain management, and to present a practical primary care framework for guiding treatment decisions.

Setting the Stage:
Telling the Truth, With Hope

I knew by the look on her face that something was wrong. She didn't have to say it; I knew she had bad news to tell me.

He told me straight out. Sam, they found cancer. They didn't get it all.

I could tell by the way the nurses kept coming in and out of the room and looking at the baby that something was wrong. But where was my doctor, all that time? How come they didn't explain to us what they were worried about?

Hospice teaches that people do better with the truth. They can mobilize personal resources if they know what they are up against. Studies on communities under siege during World War II demonstrated that those that were told the truth coped far more effectively than those that were not given the facts. Individuals and the people who love them invent their own explanations and become deeply suspicious of care providers if there is failure to communicate.

Dying patients deprived of truth are deprived of opportunities for healing. Family members and close friends can be great sources of support, but they need guidance to know how to be helpful. Family members need to hear the truth clearly, ideally when the patient is present. The personal physician can model a gentle, open, straightforward approach to the situation. She or he can offer permission for all to share emotional pain, to ask questions, and a chance to agree on what they hope for the future. Nursing staff and ancillary personnel need information about the diagnosis, prognosis, and treatment plan. They need to know how much the patient and family understand and how open they are to talking about it.

Conferences attended by family, the patient, and key health team members can quickly share important information, as well as provide an open, problem-solving approach to patient care issues. Conferences ought to be called at the time of initial diagnosis, at times of significant change in the patient's status, and before transition to another institution, hospice, or home. Some physicians can comfortably conduct these meetings; others prefer to let an experienced team player, perhaps a chaplain or social worker, conduct the meeting, freeing the physician to answer overt questions and notice those asked nonverbally.

It is important to attend to issues of confidentiality in family conferences. That which the family shares "publicly" is acceptable grist for conversation in a family meeting. That which is discussed privately with the doctor is not subject to family conversation, unless volunteered "publicly" within the family conference by the people involved. Staying close to the family's current understanding, such as responding to their needs, is a good, safe way to empower their growth. Pushing them to process or grieve faster doesn't work very well.

Cicely Saunders, MD, founder of the hospice movement, began her clinical work as a nurse. She trained and worked as a social worker and hospital administrator, and then studied medicine and pharmacology in order to care effectively for dying patients. She stressed the importance of truth telling, but believed that patients should be assessed individually by one who knew them well. She says:

> It is not right to deliberately deceive . . . I do not, however, think it is essential for every patient to know he is dying. . . . The most important principle is love; not sentimentality, but compassion and understanding. Those who establish close contact with their patients will best be able to decide whether they want or need to be enlightened and will approach as friends with courtesy and kindness. In this setting those who want to know can accept reality and find the strength to face it.

Walking the Path:
Let the Patient Set the Pace Emotionally

Elizabeth Kübler-Ross, MD, has contributed enormously to our understanding of the dying process by labeling emotional stages experienced at the end of life: denial, anger, bargaining, depression, and acceptance. These unpredictable components occur and reoccur as people experience end-of-life realities. Too often, busy clinicians have tried to encourage patients to move on to another "stage." It is better to simply be with patients in whatever stage or combination of emotional stages they are in at the time. This requires slowing down. We cannot make it happen, but we can allow it to happen, often in a short space of time.

Respecting the rich life experience the patient brings, the doctor can gently remind the patient of the strength that has been used in overcoming other life circumstances (job loss, failed marriages, etc). Hope is possible even in difficult times.

Self-Determination:
Establish a Road Map for the Future

The best person to decide limits of treatment is the patient, in open consultation with key others (loved ones, perhaps spiritual guides, lawyers). The best time to begin thinking about those decisions is when the patient is functionally competent and understands the facts about the situation, including the uncertainty always inherent in medical judgments. Establishing informed consent includes helping patients access and understand the information they need to make an informed choice that best fits their unique situation. Ideally, family members also hear and understand these decisions, and can support the patient in the process.

Failure to make a plan for end-of-life treatments is fraught with difficulty. Planning should begin as soon as the patient has recovered from the emotional shock of hearing the truth about the diagnosis. Ideally, all patients should talk with their doctors and families about how they wish to be cared for at the end of life. But, unfortunately in our death-denying American culture, most do not do so until serious illness strikes.

The federal Right of Self Determination Act passed in December 1991 assigns institutions the responsibility to inform patients of their opportunities to limit health care treatment options. Nursing homes, hospitals, clinics, and health maintenance organizations must present this information to patients in written form. This information usually requires further explanation from the physician or designated nurse or social worker.

Physicians and other providers must discern the opportune moments for these conversations. This might occur when a terminally ill patient wishes to plan or when parents need to cope with a child's potentially fatal illness. Once the patient or family is motivated to think about self-determination, the physician can orchestrate the process and negotiate some of the fine points.

At every visit the physician ought to encourage the patient and family to ask questions. Not only can information be offered in response, but the patient's level of understanding can be assessed. This process of open communication and dialogue builds trust and confidence for later stages of illness.

Guidelines for Self-Determination

It is much easier to gather information during the course of medical care than in a single episode near the end of life. A specially trained nurse, chaplain, discharge planner, or social worker can collect this important information for the physician.

1. Identify key people (family, friends, etc.). List in the chart the names and phone numbers of people who ought to be involved and informed. Note their relationship to the patient (e.g., daughter, nephew, neighbor). Note special circumstances such as former mates or estranged children. Indicate how these people are to be included.

2. Identify a spiritual framework or religious affiliation. Note the names and phone numbers of ministers, priests, or spiritual guides who ought to be involved. Note specific rituals and who will arrange for them.

3. Identify a proxy or person with durable power of attorney. Indicate whether he or she can make health care decisions if the patient cannot. Note if a will has been written, and if the proxy or family can access important documents (insurance papers, etc.).

4. List people and resources available for end-of-life care. Most people die in hospitals or institutions. Ask patients where they prefer to die. If it is at home, describe the physical adjustments that can be made (e.g., hospital bed set up in dining room near ground floor bathroom).

5. Identify values and philosophy of life. Briefly describe the patient's view of life. Indicate how the patient would prioritize quality of life (symptom free and alert), ability to communicate with family and friends, and freedom from pain. Ask directly whether it would be preferable to live longer if this meant a bit more pain, or live less long if this meant less pain. Ask how important it is for the patient to make health care decisions. Assess the patient's trust and confidence in the health care system and primary doctor. Patients who have had difficult experiences with physicians, institutional insensitivity, or third-party payers may find it difficult to trust a health care team.

6. Ask about unfinished business. Ask what the patient wishes to accomplish before death (e.g., people they wish to see or call, or old business to finish).

7. Explore the attitudes toward technology to prolong life. Using descriptions, ask if the patient and family wish the following:

  a. renal dialysis, if the kidneys stop working.

  b. intubation, if breathing stops briefly.

  c. ventilator, if breathing does not resume quickly.

  d. feeding tube, if unable to eat by mouth.

  e. central intravenous line, if unable to drink.

  f. cardiac massage, if the heart stops working.

If any of these are indicated but not available locally, ask if the patient prefers to go to another facility to receive it. Consider transfer implications on family visits, religious support, and new physician rapport.

8. Ask if antibiotics, parenteral nutrition, and other IV medications ought to be used during the last days of life.

9. If feasible, does the patient desire organ donation?

Advance directives, living wills, or written guidelines for end-of-life treatment are extremely useful documents. To be done well, the process requires a sensitive and skilled interviewer who can engage patients at a level of imagination and degree of life planning that may be new to them. Often the questions need to be asked several times, and perhaps by several people to help the patient find a clear answer. As circumstances change, patients and families will revisit and rethink these concepts in light of specific needs. The process of decision making is one of co-creation between patient, physician, health care team, and family within the context of institutional guidelines and community standards. Conflict and differences of opinion are inevitable.

Family conferences can be a useful technique to refocus those involved on the real needs of the patient, and diffuse bickering about specific choices. If the conflict does not yield to these simple measures, consultation is often available from ethics committees, hospice organizations, or social workers and mental health workers trained in family dynamics.

Opening the System:
Involving Family and Consultants

Intensive therapies are often necessary near the end of life. The personal physician ought to anticipate for the patient and family the role and style of the intensivists. Surgeons, chemotherapists, and radiation therapists all come in varying manners and bedside styles. Patients can be coached to ask questions and to seek a more informed role in their care if they know that the personal physician expects this of them. The consultant has specific information about particular forms of therapy, and it is appropriate for the personal physician to inform the patient that part of the consultant's role is educational. Patients who are more actively involved in their care appear to do better.

The family physician can learn how well particular consultants convey understandable information by asking what the patient understands. As coordinator and sometimes "quarterback," the personal physician is very important. Choices among alternative therapies ought to be consistent with the patient's wishes. If following the patient's wishes is outside the moral code of the primary physician or the consultant, another physician ought to be sought. Often this can be a partner or a primary care colleague.

The process of terminal illness profoundly affects the families involved. There is a shift in usual patterns of living as others assume the roles previously assumed by the ill person. Flexible, resourceful families with a range of coping styles can accommodate these changes with stress. If they receive reasonable support they can emerge from a terminal illness with a sense of satisfaction at a difficult job well done. Rigid, already stressed, and fractured families will have great difficulty coping with yet another insurmountable problem.

Hospital routines can be profoundly upsetting to those not yet familiar with Western medicine. For example, an Asian family found it very disturbing to have their child's blood drawn repeatedly in the hospital. They nearly left against medical advice. A respected elder Asian man and a young bilingual interpreter helped negotiate a compromise. Blood drawing was kept to a minimum. Experienced outsiders such as ministers or respected elders can be invaluable in framing medical advice in a culturally acceptable manner.

A Native American family found it spiritually healing to include native healers among those caring for a young woman with metastatic cancer. Their physician wisely authorized the burning of sage and use of tobacco for her care in the hospital.

Families can be coached to apply their innate coping skills and practical wisdom in the foreign territory of the hospital. The remarkable coping that occurs routinely among many families can be a source of strength when terminal illness strikes. In all institutions there are inadvertent mishaps. IVs get placed poorly, lines come out, busy nurses are slow to answer call lights. Families can learn to extend the patient's energy in asking the system for what they need, and feel useful in the process.

Families should be counseled to access help and manage patient concerns after hours. Emergency medical service (EMS) teams have well-established, effective protocols for response. It is wise to anticipate for families the consequences of calling them to the scene. EMS teams are often obliged to follow protocols rather than family or patient preferences in an emergency.

It is the responsibility of the primary care physician to document the treatment plan clearly in the medical record so that it can be followed after hours by an on-call physician. The patient's current resuscitation status and end-of-life documents ought to be in the office chart and available in hospitals likely to be used.

Negotiate Conflict:
See the Big Picture

Intensivist consultants offer their own perspective. Experienced nurses have strong opinions. The wise primary physician listens to the tune played by the orchestra of care providers and lets it play if the patient is well served. Intervention is necessary if conflict or differences of opinion hamper patient care. Sometimes the physician can mediate disputes; sometimes chaplains or patient advocates can serve this role. The referee should stay close to family values and educate all concerned to the imperfect, regimented community of the hospital. Mediators need to look widely for cooperation and compromise among patient, family members, health care system, and cultural heritage. Physicians should avoid small-thinking consultants and insist on organizational tolerance for each patient's definition of family and religion.

Recently, in a hospital that prides itself on compassion, a frightened lesbian patient was admitted for minor surgery. She requested that her best friend and partner be allowed to visit her. The charge nurse declined and moved her to another room for fear that other patients would be offended by one woman offering comfort to another woman. The head nurse, a wise woman of experience, found it possible to view the patient's partner as family. The humiliation the patient endured was at least addressed when she was offered an apology by the hospital.

Total Pain Management

Cicely Saunders, MD, used the term *total pain* to mean all the patient suffers, including noxious physical symptoms. Components of emotional, social, bureaucratic, financial, and spiritual angst contribute to this pain burden. Primary care physicians are ideal managers of this wide range of issues. A useful treatment approach is Jack Annon's PLISSIT model. The acronym stands for **permission, limited information, specific suggestions,** and **intensive therapy.** All primary care physicians should offer **permission** to patients and their families to find help, to share emotion and pain, and to move at their own pace in the process. Patients and families need **limited information** in a form they can use and understand about the **specifics** of their illnesses and the context of their situations.

Doctors ought to offer **specific suggestions** for symptom control. Prevention of bed sores, continence management, and relief of pain and constipation are part of maintaining human dignity and hence essential in relieving suffering. Primary care physicians usually orchestrate others to provide **intensive therapy** such as surgery, chemotherapy, or family counseling. They may also appropriately consult hospice units, ethics committees, or pain centers.

Physical Pain Management

Although it is artificial to discuss physical pain apart from the person who experiences it, some generalizations can be made.

1. Estimate how long the patient has to live. Gravely ill patients may live for weeks; actively dying patients are likely to die in 72 hours.
2. Assess symptomatic factors and treat each with appropriate therapies. Use nonnarcotic analgesia initially.
3. Continually reassess pain status. Consult with the patient, nurses, and family as to adequacy of pain relief. Escalate to narcotic analgesia promptly when indicated. Limit the dose for disagreeable side effects or patient preference. Document the rationale in the chart.
4. Think about pharmacokinetics principles. Do not increase the morphine dose before peak analgesia is achieved from the previous dose. Remember that cancer patients can have increased metabolism of drugs; patients in renal or hepatic failure may have very slow drug metabolism.

Emotional Pain:
Anticipatory Grief Management

Early in the dying process, after recovery from the shock of terminal diagnosis, many patients and families begin to notice the future they will not have. They imaginatively recognize that they may not live to see a child grow up, or get a promotion, or go on next season's fishing trip. The family may begin to grieve for the lost adulthood of their dying child. Death is very far away, but a gray cloud of sadness falls. Others express their anger openly, finding fault endlessly. Care providers may get the brunt of their anger.

Personal physicians can help by seeing the patient regularly, looking for opportunities to help patients and involved others express emotional pain, as well as to find symptomatic relief of physical symptoms. It is a mistake to take away denial. Patients use it productively to return to meaningful work, and escape emotional turmoil for a time. Dying patients have limited time and they ought to be helped to live intentionally.

This can be a time of personal growth, with a deepening of family intimacy. It is also a time of painful realization that some friends and family cannot stand the truth. Many people will chose to avoid the subject of illness, choosing a false bravado instead. The physician's willingness to engage in plain talk can be a relief. It is important to offer clear invitations to speak openly, but to allow the patient and circumstances to set the pace.

A formerly vigorous professor sought terminal care from a young internist following his diagnosis of a rapidly growing brain tumor. Despite his increasing aphasia and frailty, his wife helped him maintain a satisfying quiet life at home. Old friends often stopped by their gracious home for late afternoon tea and conversation. He had few physical symptoms. His physician suggested return visits at 3-month intervals, unless symptoms arose. His wife felt abandoned, as maintaining the home was exhausting, and the visitors were a mixed blessing. At the 3-month appointment, the physician discerned the wife's fatigue, but too quickly suggested nursing home placement as a solution. Feeling angry, and misunderstood, the wife nearly fired the doctor.

Had the physician understood that her role must include helping the wife express her needs as well as those of the patient, much of this unhappiness could have been avoided. Helping the wife to think through options might have included consideration of nursing home respite care. Had the wife been given more permission to tell her story, she may have come to trust that both she and the physician had her husband's best interest at heart.

Actively Dying:
Letting Go of Life

As patients near the end of life, they *appear* to need less from their physicians. Still, it is a mistake for the doctor to visit less regularly.

Although the patient relinquishes decision making to caregivers and begins to tune out on the business of living, he or she should not be abandoned. The doctor does important modeling for the family and the health care team by continuing to see the patient. The focus of the visits changes as pain relief is assured, symptoms are managed, and there is little energy for conversation. The family and the health care team may become those most served by the visit.

The caregiver needs physician support in assuming an increased and ever-changing role. He or she is actively grieving life changes and inevitable losses. Dying can take an exhaustingly long time. Even after mastering this role, the caregiver may still need help in letting professionals come into the home or transfer the patient to a nursing home, hospital, or hospice. Commonly caregivers cannot plan beyond the death for the next phase of life.

These principles of grief management apply to family and caregivers, as well as to patients. Allow the caregivers to be where they are. Do not push. Be available in a quiet accepting way.

It is also important to remember that the physician is grieving the loss of the dying patient. Too frequently doctors deny difficult feelings or push themselves to work harder when they feel stressed or unsure about what to do. Doctors' families and office staffs sustain the effects of these behaviors (e.g., short, irritated responses, lack of energy for family activities). More useful coping strategies include requesting supervision from an experienced, objective colleague or mental health professional. Often by sharing the facts of the case and the feelings it elicits the next steps become clear. Do not do it all alone. Use partners, colleagues, friends, family, and recreation to keep your own personal balance.

Physicians appropriately vary in their decisions to attend patients' funerals. Seeing family members in the office soon after the patient's death is clearly helpful. Questions can be answered, support given, and anticipatory guidance offered on the grief work that lies ahead.

Talking about the person who has died helps process the emotional pain of the experience. Friends and neighbors may say nothing, leaving the grieving one with the unhappy choice of feeling lonely or initiating conversation about the subject. Those willing to share grief may mistakenly encourage the bereaved person to feel better, faster. The physician can help by coaching the bereaved person through these difficult times, remembering that anniversaries (birthdays, holidays, death date) will reawaken grief, perhaps for years.

Do not rush to push the person out of their pain. Let it be. The miracle of healing can occur if the pain is allowed in the company of a gentle guide who is not afraid of the emotion shared.

Honest belief in the person's capacity to survive and even grow from the grief can be life preserver enough for growth and healing. Words and explanations are not very useful. Honest answering of questions, sitting quietly, and attentive listening are golden expressions of genuine faith in the other.

Summary

The management of the dying process through active collaboration between patient, family, and health care team is best done by a primary care physician who understands the concept and treatment of total pain. These principles apply to other less intense loss experiences such chronic illness, loss of an eye, loss of a job, loss of reputation. The relationship and procedural and organizational skills necessary are within the scope of primary care physicians.

Recommended Reading

Bozarth-Campbell, A. R. (1982). *Life is goodbye, life is hello: Grieving well through all kinds of loss* (2nd ed.). Minneapolis, MN: CompCare Publications.
Kübler-Ross, E. (1987). *AIDS, The ultimate challenge.* New York: Macmillan.
Morris, D. B. (1991). *The culture of pain.* Berkeley: University of California Press.
Walsh, M., & McGoldrick, H. (1991). *Living beyond loss.* New York: Norton.

17
■ ■ ■

Health Maintenance in Clinical Practice:

Strategies and Barriers

PAUL S. FRAME

Introduction

Obstacles to the implementation of preventive services in clinical practice include barriers raised by patients, physicians, and the health care delivery system itself. Physicians may overcome these barriers to a great extent by improving their time management skills, practice organization systems, and reinforcement mechanisms. For clinical prevention to be successfully initiated and maintained in practice, the program must be simple and include only procedures the providers believe are worthwhile; an organized record system should be used; a system of checks and reinforcements for prevention must be instituted in the practice routine; and adequate time for preventive services must be allocated, either by using paramedical personnel or by restricting the practice size.

During the past decade, the concept that selective health maintenance procedures should be offered to all patients at appropriate intervals has replaced the once widely recommended but scientifically unsubstantiated theory that all adults should have a complete physical examination annually. The specific diseases screened for in a health maintenance program should meet screening criteria similar to those shown in Table 17.1. Failure to fulfill each one of these criteria means that screening is unlikely to be beneficial.

AUTHOR'S NOTE: Adapted from "Health Maintenance in Clinical Practice: Strategies and Barriers" by Paul S. Frame, 1992, *American Family Physician, 45,* 1192-1200. Used with permission of the American Academy of Family Physicians.

Table 17.1 Screening Criteria for Health Maintenance Interventions

1. The condition must have a significant effect on the quality or quantity of life.

2. Acceptable methods of treatment must be available.

3. The condition must have an asymptomatic period during which detection and treatment significantly reduce morbidity and/or mortality.

4. Treatment in the asymptomatic phase must yield a therapeutic result superior to that obtained by delaying treatment until symptoms appear.

5. Tests that are acceptable to patients must be available at reasonable cost for detection of the condition in the asymptomatic period.

6. The incidence of the condition must be sufficient to justify the cost of screening.

Specific preventive care recommendations for asymptomatic adults have been made by a number of authors and organizations, including the Canadian Task Force on the Periodic Health Examination (1979), the American Cancer Society (Eddy, 1980), and, most recently, the U.S. Preventive Services Task Force (1989). Although these recommendations vary significantly, a core of agreement can be found: that all adults should be screened for cardiovascular risk factors, tobacco use, hypertension, and hyperlipidemia; that women over 50 years of age should be screened for breast cancer; that all women should be screened for cervical cancer; and that all adults should be given a tetanus booster every 10 years. Screening for colon cancer is also recommended by many, although the evidence in support of this intervention is less compelling.

Numerous studies have shown that primary care physicians are not offering this core group of recommended procedures to many of their patients. Survey studies indicate that physicians think they provide more health maintenance than audits of actual performance demonstrate (Woo, Woo, Cook, Weisberg, & Goldman, 1985). Furthermore, patients in higher socioeconomic groups and health-conscious, low-risk patients are those most likely to receive health maintenance care.

This chapter explains some of the barriers to implementation of a health maintenance program in primary care practice and discusses strategies that can help physicians attain the goal of providing selective longitudinal health maintenance to all patients.

Table 17.2 Barriers to Clinical Prevention

HEALTH SYSTEM BARRIERS

     Inadequate reimbursement
     Lack of health insurance
     Population mobility
     Patients with multiple physicians
     Categoric, sporadic screening programs (e.g., health fairs)

PATIENT BARRIERS

     Ignorance of screening benefits
     Doubts about the physician's ability to detect a hidden disease
     Cost of screening procedures
     Discomfort
     A conscious or unconscious desire not to change unhealthy habits

PHYSICIAN BARRIERS

     Uncertainty about conflicting recommendations
     Uncertainty about the value of screening tests
     Disorganized medical records
     Delayed and indirect gratification from screening
     Lack of time

Barriers to Clinical Prevention

Barriers to clinical prevention can be categorized as physician, patient, and health system barriers (Table 17.2). Some of these barriers can be influenced by physicians in the practice setting, but others are beyond physician control. Several barriers overlap categories. For example, inadequate knowledge of the benefits of screening can be a factor with both patients and physicians. After hearing for decades that an annual physical examination is necessary for asymptomatic patients, complete with electrocardiogram, chest radiographs, and multiple blood tests, both physicians and patients are now confused about which procedures are truly worthwhile. However, authoritative sources such as the *Guide to Clinical Preventive Services*, from the U.S. Preventive Services Task Force, and persistent physician and patient education should decrease any skepticism about the value of the core group of health maintenance procedures.

Health System Barriers

Lack of reimbursement for preventive procedures is a medical system barrier that affects both patients and physicians. Third-party payers for health care justifiably have been reluctant to pay for unproven preventive procedures that could potentially be applied to entire populations. However, the core of proven preventive procedures is not large and, with the exception of mammography, the tests are not expensive. The INSURE project (1987) demonstrated the feasibility of reimbursement in such instances.

The fact that large numbers of adults have no health insurance at all is a major barrier to health maintenance. Uninsured persons are more likely to be inactive patients or to have no primary care physician, and they are at higher risk than the general population for preventable disease.

Fragmentation of health care may be considered an urban issue. However, patient mobility, public health clinics, and emergency patients may result in fragmentation even in rural settings. In this situation, it is often not clear which provider is responsible for health maintenance.

Population mobility is a significant barrier to clinical prevention. The author's practice is in an apparently stable rural area, yet there is a 17% annual turnover in the practice population. To deal with population mobility, strategies must be developed that encourage patients to share to a significant degree the responsibility for their own health maintenance. Patient handouts such as the one shown in Figure 17.1 can emphasize this shared responsibility. An owner's manual for the human body, similar to an automobile owner's manual, has been developed (Deming, 1989), and others have developed patient health diaries that contain a health maintenance flow sheet, similar to the immunization record parents keep for their children. The patient is responsible for keeping it current. At a more sophisticated level, computer "smart" cards store similar information. The responsibility for health maintenance must be shared by patients and primary care physicians.

Screening health fairs sponsored by diverse organizations such as hospitals, service clubs, and churches merely fragment health maintenance and probably do more harm than good (Berwick, 1985). Frequently, inappropriate tests are offered that do not meet screening criteria, or the tests focus on only one organ system, or do not

HEALTH IS YOUR RESPONSIBILITY

Your lifestyle and habits determine to a large degree whether you will be healthy or will be at high risk for serious illness and accidents. Only you can decide if you will lead a healthy or destructive lifestyle.

SOME IMPORTANT ACTIONS YOU CAN TAKE INCLUDE:

1. Do not smoke tobacco.

2. Wear seatbelts whenever you ride in an automobile.

3. Drink alcohol in moderation, if at all, and never drive when you have been drinking.

4. Exercise regularly.

5. Be aware of the stresses and tensions in your life. Reduce non-essential stress.

Tri-County Family Medicine has a health maintenance program we want everyone involved in. You should have a complete physical examination when you first come to Tri-County and also, of course, if you are not feeling well or have a medical problem.

The focus of our health maintenance program, however, is on periodic checkups for a few specific diseases by tests of proven value. For most people this will mean a checkup every two years if you are under age 50 and every year for those over age 50. The complete program is shown on the back of this page.

CERTAIN PROBLEMS REQUIRE YOUR COOPERATION AT HOME

1. If you are overweight, now is the best time to start a diet.

2. Check regularly for new lumps, especially in the mouth, neck and groin. Report these to your doctor if they persist more than one month.

3. WOMEN: A. Check your breasts for lumps every month.
B. Report vaginal bleeding after menopause.

4. MEN: Check for lumps in the testicles.

> ### TRI-COUNTY FAMILY MEDICINE PROGRAM

Red Jacket Street Dansville, N.Y. 14437 (716) 335-6041	Park Avenue Cohocton, N.Y. 14826 (716) 384-5310	61 State Street Nunda, N.Y. 14517 (716) 468-2528	North Church Street Canaseraga, N.Y. 14822 (607) 545-8333	East Naples Street Wayland, N.Y. 14572 (716) 728-5131

Figure 17.1. Patient Health Maintenance Handout

provide rational health maintenance for that particular person. Usually no provision for repeat testing at defined intervals is offered. Follow-up of abnormal results may be nonexistent, and normal results may falsely reassure people at risk. For example, a sedentary smoker with a family history of heart disease may feel he is "OK" if his cholesterol level is normal. Too often, the unstated primary purpose of such health fairs is really promotion of the sponsoring organization.

Patient Barriers

The adage "If it ain't broke, don't fix it" may partly explain patient reluctance to request health maintenance procedures. Patients who feel well see little need to spend money for uncomfortable procedures that will probably have normal results. In addition, a conscious or unconscious desire not to give up unhealthy habits is also a patient barrier to health maintenance. Smokers are among the patients least compliant with health maintenance procedures.

Physician Barriers

An effective preventive program does not happen by itself; it requires a commitment to health maintenance by the physician and the practice, including nurses and support staff. Health maintenance activities should be a priority, not just an option to be included if time allows. The commitment must be maintained on an ongoing basis.

Providing health maintenance for all patients is difficult and time-consuming. A program that includes only the minimum of procedures may at first seem insufficient but may actually prove to be a major daily commitment for the physician. At every patient visit, the question must be asked: "Is this patient's health maintenance up to date?"

Strategies for Implementing Prevention

The first step in implementing a preventive program is to decide which procedures are worthwhile. Recommendations from the Canadian Task Force on the Periodic Health Examination, the American Cancer Society, and the U.S. Preventive Services Task Force can be helpful in this process. A basic core group of interventions should be selected. Physicians who feel strongly about performing additional tests or testing at more frequent intervals should feel free to do so, but the core practice protocol should be kept as concise as possible.

ADULT HEALTH MAINTENANCE

AGE:	18	19	20	21	22	23	24	25	26	27	28	29	30	31	32	33	34	35	36	37	38	39	40	41	42	43	44	45	46	47	48	49
DATE:																																
Complete H.&P.			once at entry																													
Hx Rheumatic Fever			once at entry																													
Hx Smoking	•		•										•										•									
Hx Alcohol Use	•		•						•				•						•				•						•			
Blood Pressure	•		•		•		•		•		•		•		•		•		•		•		•		•		•		•		•	
Weight	•		•						•				•						•				•						•			
Pap Test	•		•		•		•		•		•		•		•		•		•		•		•		•		•		•		•	
Breast Exam	•		•		•		•		•		•		•		•		•		•		•		•		•		•		•		•	
Cholestrol			•				•				•				•				•				•				•				•	
Stool Occult Blood																							•		•		•		•		•	
Education																																
Seat Belts	•		•										•										•									
Teach Self-Palpation Breast, Neck, Testes			•										•										•									
Teach Report Post-Menopausal Bleeding																																
Teach Report Mouth and Skin Lesions																							•									

AGE:	50	51	52	53	54	55	56	57	58	59	60	61	62	63	64	65	66	67	68	69	70	71	72	73	74	75	76	77	78	79	80
DATE:	2-86	3-87	2-88	3-90																											
Complete H.&P.	\ once at entry																														
Hx Rheumatic Fever	\ once at entry																														
Hx Smoking QUIT	X										•										•										
Hx Alcohol Use	/					•					•					•					•								•		
Blood Pressure	/		/		/		•		•		•		•		•		•		•		•		•		•		•		•		•
Weight	/					•					•					•					•					•					•
Pap Test	E		N		Hysterectomy 1987																										
Breast Exam	E	E	E	/	/	•	•	•	•	•	•	•	•	•	•	•	•	•	•	•	•	•	•	•	•	•	•	•	•	•	•
Cholestrol			/				•				•				•																
Stool Occult Blood	R	R	/	/	/	•	•	•	•	•	•	•	•	•	•	•	•	•	•	•	•	•	•	•	•	•	•	•	•	•	•
Education																															
Seat Belts	/										•										•										
Teach Self-Palpation Breast, Neck, Testes	/										•										•										
Teach Report Post-Menopausal Bleeding	/	N									•										•										
Teach Report Mouth and Skin Lesions	/										•										•										
Mammogram	E	E	E	\	\																										

JCM 477:08

Figure 17.2. Example of a Patient Maintenance Flow Sheet

NOTE: Symbols used: / = test performed, result normal; X = test performed, result abnormal; R = patient refused test; E = test performed elsewhere; N = test not indicated.

Health Maintenance Flow Sheet

A flow sheet is the most commonly used tool for tracking health maintenance in practice (Figure 17.2). Studies have shown that flow sheets improve physician compliance with health maintenance, although physicians perform more health maintenance services than they record on the flow sheet. A flow sheet alone—without a reinforcement system—does not result in acceptable levels of compliance.

The flow sheet must be brief—a maximum of one page. It should be organized so that the dates of health maintenance procedures can be seen at a glance. It should require a minimum of writing by the provider, utilizing codes and letters instead of words. It should extend at least to age 80 and should provide extra lines at the bottom so that additional tests can be added and the flow sheet can be individualized for each patient. The flow sheet should be placed prominently in the chart, preferably on the front cover, to facilitate frequent use and easy review of the patient's health maintenance status.

Establishing a flow sheet-based tracking system for health maintenance requires a large initial investment of time and energy by the practice members. Flow sheets and data bases must be established for all patients, and because the concepts are new, they require education for patients, physicians, and staff. The process becomes easier after everyone is familiar with the system and data bases and flow sheets have been established for most patients. With time, the physician begins to see success, as measured by the reduction of risk factors, changes in unhealthy behaviors, and the detection of early curable disease.

Continuity of care is a necessary element for reinforcing physician motivation for health maintenance. If physicians do not care for the same patients over time, they will not experience a reward from the initial investment in health maintenance and will be much less likely to continue it. Without continuity of care, the physician is less likely to feel responsible for the patient's welfare and less likely to experience a sense of failure if the patient contracts a preventable disease.

Example of a System

Figure 17.2 shows an example of a health maintenance flow sheet; This form is used by the author. The month and year are placed at the top of each column. Multiple entry codes, as illustrated in this flow sheet, keep the physician apprised of the status of each health maintenance procedure. Simple "yes/no" coding does not give adequate information about the range of possible situations. The physician can add notes at the bottom of the flow sheet about a patient's particular situation.

On a patient's first visit, an attempt is made to obtain a data base, preferably through a complete physical examination. This examination is fairly traditional, including a past history, family history, and social history, in addition to a head-to-toe physical examination. If the patient is asymptomatic, the only tests performed are those indicated by the flow sheet. Chest radiograph, electrocardiogram, blood chemistry profile, complete blood count, and urinalysis are not routine parts of this examination, unless indicated by clinical symptoms or signs. If the patient remains asymptomatic, this data-base examination is the only time the patient is asked to undergo a complete physical examination. A review of the components of a physical examination that are worth including for asymptomatic patients has been published recently (Oberler & LaForce, 1989).

At the end of the initial examination, the physician discusses acute problems with the patient and formulates an individual problem list. At this time, the patient is given a copy of the health maintenance handout (Figure 17.1) and an informal risk analysis is made. The patient is informed about which health maintenance procedures are indicated at the time and is requested to return for a health maintenance check-up (not a complete physical examination) at the appropriate interval according to the flow-sheet protocol. The next visit is usually in 1 or 2 years, depending on the patient's age. The completed flow sheet allows the provider to tell at a glance at each patient visit whether health maintenance is up to date and which specific procedures are indicated. Some practices use a computerized health risk appraisal, such as the one created by the Carter Center of Emory University (1987) in conjunction with the Centers for Disease Control and Prevention, to assist and add impact to the initial risk evaluation.

The health maintenance handout is purposefully brief. The front side (Figure 17.1) emphasizes patient responsibilities and lifestyle habits that only the patient can change. The reverse side of the handout includes a copy of the flow sheet for use by the more motivated patients.

A postcard reminder system prompts patients who do not have appointments for acute problems to return for health maintenance. A file is maintained in each office, divided into months and extending at least 2 years into the future. When the physician wishes to initiate a prompt, "RV ____ years, send card" is written at the top of the encounter form. Some computer billing systems allow this to be done through the billing system.

This type of manual health maintenance tracking system can work well for active patients if the physician is motivated. The major weaknesses of a manual system are dependence on physician motivation and inadequate outreach to inactive patients.

Computerized Systems

To be cost-effective, a computerized health maintenance tracking system must be linked to the practice's billing system, so that demographic data entry does not have to be duplicated and health maintenance procedures can be entered into the record quickly. Multiple entry options, similar to those described for the manual system, must be available, and it must be possible to designate whether and when reminders are to be sent, regardless of whether the patient makes an appointment.

Time Management

The most important barrier to physician implementation of health maintenance is lack of time. Performing only proven health maintenance procedures and keeping an organized record system will save time, but these steps alone may not be enough. Paramedical personnel, physician assistants, and nurse practitioners can be very helpful. Physician assistants can provide continuity for many patients and offer health maintenance as part of their job. Nurses and clerical office personnel can also play a major role in achieving health maintenance goals, if they have enough time to do so. Positive reinforcement for a job well done will help to encourage staff commitment.

Behavior Reinforcement

If health maintenance is to be an integral part of the practice, some mechanism for reinforcing and rewarding compliance must be built into the system and used on a regular basis. One such mechanism is periodic audits of health maintenance performance with peer review. Such audits do not have to be lengthy. A secretary can retrieve charts of patients seen on a given day, or a random sample of a small number of charts from each physician can be selected for audit by another physician, physician assistant, or nurse. Whatever the mechanism, it should be ongoing and incorporated into practice routines. Audit analysis also allows the practice members to evaluate whether all procedures in the protocol are considered worthwhile. If not, the test should be removed from the protocol.

Summary

Rational health maintenance is a cornerstone of primary care and should be provided to all patients. Implementing health maintenance in practice requires motivation and a structured approach, including: relying on worthwhile interventions, keeping the program simple, maintaining an organized record system that includes a reminder protocol, managing time effectively, and providing a reinforcement mechanism to maintain compliance.

References

Berwick, D. M. (1985). Screening in health fairs. A critical review of benefits, risks, and costs. *Journal of the American Medical Association, 254,* 1492-1498.

Canadian Task Force on the Periodic Health Examination. (1979). The periodic health examination. *Canadian Medical Association Journal, 121,* 1193-1254.

Deming, J. (1989). *Owner's maintenance handbook for humans.* Elm Grove: Wisconsin Academy of Family Physicians.

Eddy, D. (1980). ACS report on the cancer-related health checkup. *CA, 30,* 193-240.

INSURE Project. (1987). *Final report.* Menlo Park, CA: Henry J. Kaiser Family Foundation.

Oberler, S. K., & LaForce, F. M. (1989). The periodic physical examination in asymptomatic adults. *Annals of Internal Medicine, 110,* 214-226.

The Carter Center of Emory University. (1987). *Health risk appraisal program.* Decatur, GA: Carter Center of Emory University.

U.S. Preventive Services Task Force. (1989). *Guide to clinical preventive services.* Baltimore, MD: Williams & Wilkins.

Woo, B., Woo, B., Cook, E. F., Weisberg, M., & Goldman, L. (1985). Screening procedures in the asymptomatic adult. Comparison of physicians' recommendations, patients' desires, published guidelines, and actual practice. *Journal of the American Medical Association, 254,* 1480-1484.

18
■ ■ ■

Patient Education
in the Rural Practice

PATRICIA A. GIBSON

CLAUDIA J. KAPP

Introduction

Patient education is "a process of influencing patient behavior, producing changes in knowledge, attitudes and skills required to maintain or improve health" (National Task Force on Training Family Physicians in Patient Education, 1979). Patient education is an integral part of any primary care practice, rural or urban. The physician draws on his or her clinical knowledge and rapport with the patient and provides leadership, involving the entire office staff in the patient education program. Essential to any effective patient education program is determining patients' needs and locating, evaluating, and utilizing appropriate resources. This chapter will cover these overriding principles.

Scarcity of health manpower, monetary constraints, and lack of easy access to patient education materials in the rural setting may make it more difficult to develop an effective patient education program. However, the rural setting also provides a number of opportunities for the health care provider and the consumer. A small number of people with a common goal can make a significant impact on health in the community. Administratively, patient education efforts can be more easily coordinated in a smaller organization. Smaller practices have less inertia and fewer layers of bureaucracy, allowing for creativity and innovation. Launching a patient education campaign in a rural practice provides a framework for team building, shared responsibility, and personal and professional growth.

Rural health care providers are keenly aware of the need for extension of services and the importance of avoiding duplication. Patient education provides a unique opportunity for health care professionals and other community resources to form partnerships for improved health in the community.

Rationale for Patient Education

Patient education goes on in the office, whether or not the physician and staff consciously teach. The receptionist provides patient education in scheduling appointments or doing telephone triage. Nurses and laboratory and X-ray personnel inform patients about treatment, procedures, and tests. Clerical staff provide information about billing and insurance and communicate administrative philosophy. Office staff can encourage browsing through patient education materials and are in a position to receive negative feedback patients may be reluctant to give the doctor. Should patient education continue unguided and unstructured or should your practice develop a patient education focus in the office, utilizing the unique talents and interests of all staff members?

The pragmatist's answer is that patient education saves time and saves lives. Telling parents what kinds of reactions to expect from immunizations, or informing the person on antidepressants about the dry mouth before it happens can save telephone calls. Few physicians would consider sending a football player home from the emergency room without reminding him how to care for his freshly placed sutures. With a few simple suggestions and demonstrations, patient education can also save lives. Most primary care physicians know intuitively that more children's lives have been saved by demanding that parents use infant car seats than they will ever save in the emergency room or the intensive care unit.

For the busy physician, patient education can become a welcome break in the routine of seeing similar types of patients and problems each day. It provides a nice way to express one's creativity and to interact with patients and co-workers on a different level, without adding significant time to each encounter.

Patient education is considered an essential part of quality health care; but until recently, third-party payers did not reimburse for patient education. With the advent of the Resource Based Relative Value Scale (RBRVS), Medicare acknowledges that patient education, counseling, and coordination of care with other providers or agencies take time and effort.

Philosophy of Practice

Any effective patient education program requires commitment to patient education on the part of the entire staff. It is an integral part of every patient visit. Education must be viewed as a foundation of communication and trust between health provider and patient. An atmosphere of shared responsibility between patients and physicians allows patients to make sound choices about their health and health care (Falvo & Bosshart, 1990).

Patient Education Committee

A key element to success is a patient education committee with representatives from all departments within the practice. Inclusion of volunteers, patients, and other health care professionals with whom one works closely, such as public health nurses, social workers, pharmacists, and dietitians, can further strengthen the committee.

A patient education committee can engage in brainstorming, needs assessment, goal and priority setting, problem solving, and program evaluation. Committee membership can be added to staff job descriptions. Members' expertise and special interests can be utilized. The committee can address such questions as: "What message will be communicated? Who will provide the information? How will the message be communicated consistently? When and where will patients get information? What training or staff development is needed?" (Wytias & Jones, 1989). In a small rural practice the committee may consist of two or three members.

Table 18.1 Methods of Assessing Patients' Information Needs

1. Observe what patients read and ask about in the office.

2. Analyze the most frequent diagnoses in the practice: office setting, hospital, and emergency room.

3. Examine major causes of morbidity and mortality.

4. Consult national surveys of the core clinical content of family practice, such as that by Rosenblatt et al. (1982).

5. Survey patients: What are their major health concerns?

Assessing Needs

Effective teaching requires a learner. The information must be comprehensible and relevant to the patient's situation (Falvo, 1985). Patient education topics and materials should reflect your patient population: its demographics, including age distribution, clusters of occupations in the community, ethnic groups, educational and income levels, and health needs and interests (Table 18.1).

It is realistic to focus on a limited number of topics initially, covering acute care, chronic disease, health promotion, disease prevention and a "hot" topic (e.g., nicotine patches). Condition frequency, disease severity, potential impact of education on outcome, and health provider interest can help prioritize topics.

Applying Adult Education Research

Adult learning theory (Table 18.2) provides a helpful framework for planning an effective approach to patient education. It asserts that both the instructor and the learner are partners in the learning.

The instructor becomes a facilitator, rather than just a purveyor of information. This approach can also work with most children by providing a learning environment of mutual respect and relating subject content to the child's past experiences. Conversely, adults may need to begin as dependent learners when they enter a content

Table 18.2 Adult Learning Theory

Adult learning theory assumes that adults:

1. Become ready to learn when a real-life situation confronts and challenges them.
2. Expect to apply their learning immediately to the specific task or problem confronting them.
3. Bring many life experiences that enrich and color their learning.
4. Want to move from dependency to increased self-directedness.

area unfamiliar to them, such as diabetes management. The educator's task is to help the learner move to a more active and independent role (Knowles, 1990).

As a result of education, the patient and the family must become more independent if they are to carry out the treatment plan. As hospital stays have been shortened and chronic illnesses have become more prevalent in our society, patients and family members are being asked to assume greater responsibility for care in the home (Redman, 1988).

Patient education can improve care outcomes and lower the overall costs of health care. Patients want to be and are expected to be more active participants in their health care. If they are provided with the information and education, patients will be able to progress beyond learning facts to making judgments in daily living. Patterns of change must be reinforced if they are to become permanent, and the primary care physician is in an excellent position to sustain positive outcomes during regular follow-up visits. Providing motivation, clarification, and reinforcement of positive health behaviors and decisions takes little added time. Self-care activities can be tailored to individual patient needs, abilities, readiness to learn, coping skills, and support systems. Most patient education is provided on a one-to-one basis by the health professional, who must focus on effective communication (Table 18.3). Most of the steps in effective patient education communication are already part of the process of the physician visit: listening, observation, assessment, and recommendation.

Table 18.3 Guidelines for One-to-One Patient Education

1. Sit down to interview and counsel patients. Sitting implies caring and a willingness to spend time with the patient.

2. Recognize the "teachable moment," when the patient is receptive to new ideas and motivated to change behavior.

3. Learn the patient's priorities and involve the patient in setting learning goals.

4. Use terms the patient understands; avoid medical jargon.

5. Simplify. Present a maximum of 3 to 4 points verbally.

6. Don't overwhelm the patient with lifestyle changes. Help the patient succeed, not fail.

7. Give specific explanations and instructions; then assess the patient's understanding of the treatment plan.

8. Evaluate the patient's progress and provide positive reinforcement.

9. If the treatment plan fails, criticize the behavior, not the person.

10. Write down instructions. Written instructions increase learning retention and improve adherence (Vogt & Kapp, 1987).

Appropriate Use of
Patient Education Materials

Instructional materials alone do not constitute patient education. Patient education begins when the health professional clearly communicates information needed by the patient. Carefully selected instructional materials merely clarify, supplement, and reinforce that instruction (Falvo, 1985). The remainder of this chapter focuses on how to identify, evaluate, and use patient education materials.

Practical Implementation Considerations

In planning which resources to acquire and where to store and display them, analyze your office space and how patients move through it. For easy access, examining rooms should be equipped with frequently used materials. If one examining room is designated for children and another for obstetrical patients, appropriate models, posters, and materials may be tailored to those special needs. Blackboards are a useful teaching tool and serve to keep children busy. Informative posters on ceilings, in rest rooms, in labs and X-ray areas offer distraction and sometimes humor. A separate area within the office dedicated to patient education makes a statement to patients about the importance of patient education in the practice. It can also serve as a patient counseling area. Ideally, a mini-library could house books and audiovisuals available on loan, pamphlets, and community resource information (American Academy of Family Physicians, 1984). Materials on sensitive topics, such as AIDS, family violence, sexually transmitted diseases, and testicular self-examination, may be available in rest rooms, where patients may be more likely to take them.

Placing educational brochures and health promotion and wellness newsletters in the reception area and using a bulletin board to feature timely or seasonal health topics fosters patient learning. Educational toys such as doctor kits, educational models, and books can help allay children's fears. The magazines placed in patient areas should be carefully selected. Many magazines contain tobacco or alcohol advertisements, but an increasing number do not. Informational stickers regarding the dangers of tobacco and alcohol use can be applied over such advertisements.

The laboratory and X-ray departments, procedure rooms, and elevators are excellent sites for posters and other displays. A statement of the practice's patient education philosophy can be incorporated into a brochure that contains practical information regarding office hours, policies for handling emergencies, telephone calls, insurance, and other information about the office and staff. The brochure can also foster health promotion, disease prevention, and wellness activities.

Locating and Selecting Materials

After mapping out topics and plans for the physical display of materials, appropriate educational materials must be selected. Some common sources are listed in Table 18.4. From the myriad sources of patient education materials, it is important to select carefully those materials best suited to your practice. The physician or designated support staff should read each piece to be given to patients to ensure that it communicates the desired message and

Table 18.4 Selected Sources of Patient Education Materials

American Academy of Family
  Physicians
8880 Ward Parkway
Kansas City, MO 64114-2797

American Academy of Ophthalmology
655 Beach Street
San Francisco, CA 94109

American Academy of Pediatrics
141 Northwest Point Blvd.
P. O. Box 927
Elk Grove Village, IL 60009-0927

American Cancer Society, Inc.
777 Third Avenue
New York, NY 10027

American College of Obstetricians
  and Gynecologists
600 Maryland Avenue, Southwest
Suite 300
Washington, DC 20024-2588

American Dental Association
211 East Chicago Avenue
Chicago, IL 60611

American Diabetes Association, Inc.
National Service Center
P.O. Box 25757
1660 Duke Street
Alexandria, VA 22314

American Heart Association
7320 Greenville Avenue
Dallas, TX 75231

American Society of Hospital
  Pharmacists
4630 Montgomery Avenue
Bethesda, MD 20814

Arthritis Foundation
1314 Spring Street, Northwest
Atlanta, GA 30309

National Center for Education in
  Maternal & Child Health
38th & R Streets, Northwest
Washington, DC 20057

National Clearinghouse on Aging
330 Independence Avenue, Southwest
Washington, DC 20201

National Clearinghouse for Mental
  Health Information
Room 15C-17, Public Inquiries Sec.
5600 Fishers Lane
Rockville, MD 20857

National Diabetes Information
  Clearinghouse
Box NDIC
Bethesda, MD 20205

National Rural Health Association
301 E. Armour Blvd.
Kansas City, MO 64111

Office of Cancer Communications
NCI, Cancer Information Service
Building 31, Room 10-A-18
9000 Rockville Pike
Bethesda, MD 20205

contains no objectionable material. To evaluate patient education materials, a standardized review form (available from the author at the American Academy of Family Physicians, 1-800-274-2337) is helpful. All practice personnel can serve as reviewers. Two reviewers per piece provide balance: a health professional to assess scientific accuracy, and an office support person or trained volunteer to assure that the material is clear, understandable, and useful to the layman. An added advantage of this approach is that the entire staff becomes involved in the overall patient education effort. Pharmacists, social workers, and dietitians outside the practice can also serve as reviewers. Each brings the unique perspective of a particular area of expertise. A collaborative process can strengthen working relationships, provide a more consistent message to patients, and reduce duplication of effort.

The primary criteria in evaluating patient education materials are scientific accuracy, currency, and usefulness. Other content considerations include clear organization of ideas and appropriate scope of coverage for the intended audience. For example, if the piece is written for a newly diagnosed diabetic, does it provide the necessary explanations and instructions for self-care, without confusing and unnecessarily alarming the patient? Is the content useful and does it support the physician's objectives? Does it match the practice's usual standard of care? Does the piece contain any portions that could be perceived by patients as culturally biased, in terms of ageism, sexism, or racism? An important health message may be blocked by "putting down" a societal group to which the patient belongs.

Secondary to content is the appearance of the piece, specifically its eye-catching appeal, clarity and size of print, clarity and appropriateness of illustrations, and an adequate use of "white space." A reasonable amount of blank space is pleasing to the eye and helps emphasize ideas in the narrative. It also provides space to personalize information for a specific patient. The "perfect" pamphlet is rare, perhaps nonexistent; and so usefulness and content considerations should drive selection decisions.

Reading Level

An accurate, well-organized patient education piece will not communicate successfully if it is written at an inappropriate reading level for the intended audience. The mean reading level in the United States is between the seventh and eighth grades. Approximately 20% are functionally illiterate, reading at the fifth-grade level or below (Doak & Doak, 1980). Unfortunately, most materials designed for patients are written at a level significantly above seventh grade. The Patient's Bill of Rights and many informed consent forms are written at the college level. Various standardized scales have been developed to compute reading levels, such as the Dale Chall, the Spache, and the SMOG, which can be run manually. These scales consider word length and sentence length, and take less than 5 minutes to complete. Computerized versions of these scales are available but require the text to be typed or scanned into the computer.

Evaluative Service

The American Academy of Family Physicians Foundation (AAFP/ F) has developed a peer-review system to help family physicians select reliable, scientifically accurate materials on a wide range of clinical topics. Favorably reviewed materials are listed in the Health Education Program database, maintained by the AAFP/F's Huffington Library.

Creating Your Own Materials

Occasionally there are no suitable patient education materials available for a particular topic, or those available are too expensive. The physician can develop original materials using the same criteria of accuracy, clarity, appropriateness, and reader appeal. Using an appropriate print size, suitable white space, and paragraph headings to emphasize major points, and allowing space for personalization by the health care provider will improve any piece. Handouts covering sensitive subjects may be better received by patients in a trifold format than as a single sheet. The local print shop or newspaper office can provide layout suggestions. Finally, it is important to compute the reading level of the piece. If the piece exceeds seventh- or eighth-grade level, substitute synonyms for medical and other technical terms and shorten sentence length, emphasizing a maximum of 5 to 7 points.

Organizing Materials

After materials have been selected and obtained, they must be organized and cataloged. This may be done in various ways, such as by organ system or major topics. There are a number of classification systems available from the AAFP to use as guides. The classification must be consistent and clear to all users. The catalog can be a guide to locate less commonly used information. In the storage space a "running low" sheet placed in front of the last few pamphlets within a file provides a simple inventory control system. If this sheet contains the name of the pamphlet, name and address of its source, and cost information, pamphlets can easily be reordered. In addition, noting on the inventory control sheet the date and quantity ordered assists in future planning.

Premade Packets for Special Types of Visits

It may prove useful to prepare in advance well-organized packets for certain types of visits, such as first prenatal visits, well-baby care (age specific), obesity, or routine preventive care. Because such packets may contain a wealth of information, one should open them with the patient and make one or two specific points about the material.

Computer Software in Patient Education

The same microcomputer that is used for billing and office management can be used for a variety of patient education materials. Some computer software provides full-text patient education material as a printout (Table 18.5). Storing patient education handouts in computer format minimizes the need to invest staff time and physical space collecting, organizing, and storing brochures of various sizes and shapes. One can merely retrieve the drug or disease information needed, modify the instructions to fit the patient, and print out the piece. Although the theory is sound, the companies providing this service are still young and the material is marginal in many cases.

Beyond the Office Visit

Rural communities often call on the family physician to provide small or large group presentations. This can be done alone or in

Table 18.5 Patient Education Software

Adult Health Advisor,	Available from:
Medication Advisor,	Clinical Reference Systems, Ltd.
OB/GYN Advisor,	P.O. Box 4231
Pediatric Advisor	Englewood, CO 80155

USP Patient Drug Education Leaflet data base
12601 Twinbrook Parkway
Rockville, MD 20852

Family Practice Recertification FYPI
3 Greenwich Office Park
Greenwich, CT 06831

conjunction with other health care professionals or organizations. To merit this level of investment, a topic should be:

1. Of common interest: It needs to attract a sufficient number of people.
2. Prevalent: People should perceive a level of risk or susceptibility to stimulate a personal interest in learning about the condition.
3. Lifestyle related: The audience can be empowered to make a positive connection between their behaviors and health outcomes.
4. Improvable or changeable: Patients need hope that they can make a difference in the outcome.

It may also be useful to refer some patients for in-depth teaching to other health professionals in the community such as childbirth educators, diabetes educators, and dietitians, with reinforcement provided by the physician in follow-up visits.

Role Modeling

Regardless of which educational activities the health care provider uses, he or she also educates patients by serving as a role model. A smoke-free office makes a powerful statement to office staff and patients. Additional benefit is derived when patients perceive office staff practicing what the clinicians preach. Rural physicians are highly visible; patients see them in the grocery store, the local restaurant, or on the jogging path. Every aspect of their lifestyles, including diet, smoking, alcohol use, and seat belt use can have a profound influence on the healthy behaviors of their patients.

References

American Academy of Family Physicians. (1984). *Patient education: Home study self assessment monographs*, No. 61.

Doak, L. G., & Doak, C. C. (1980). Patient comprehension profiles: Recent findings and strategies. *Patient Counseling and Health Education, 2*(3), 101-106.

Falvo, D. R. (1985). *Effective patient education: A guide to increased compliance.* Rockville, MD: Aspen.

Falvo, D. R., & Bosshart, D. A. (1990). Patient education. In R. E. Rakel (Ed.), *Textbook of family practice* (pp. 380-389). Philadelphia, PA: W. B. Saunders.

Knowles, M. S. (1990). *The adult learner: A neglected species.* Houston, TX: Gulf.

National Task Force on Training Family Physicians in Patient Education. (1979). *Patient education: A handbook for teachers.* Kansas City, MO: Society of Teachers of Family Medicine.

Redman, B. K. (1988). *The process of patient education.* St. Louis, MO: C. V. Mosby.

Rosenblatt, R. A., Cherkin, D. C., Schneeweiss, R., Hart, L. G., Greenwald, H., Kirkwood, C. R., & Perkoff, G. T. (1982). The structure and content of family practice: Current status and future trends. *Journal of Family Practice, 25*(4), 681-722.

Vogt, H. B., & Kapp, C. (1987). Patient education in primary care practice. *Postgraduate Medicine, 81*(4), 273-278.

Wytias, C. A., & Jones, K. (1989). Engaging office staff in the education of patients. In *Proceedings of the 11th Annual Conference on Patient Education.* Kansas City, MO: Society of Teachers of Family Medicine and American Academy of Family Physicians.

Recommended Reading

Griffith, H. W. (1989). *Instructions for patients.* Philadelphia: W. B. Saunders.

Wagner, D. I., & Filak, A. (1990). Rural health promotion: An alternative delivery system. In *Proceedings of the 12th Annual Conference on Patient Education.* Kansas City, MO: Society of Teachers of Family Medicine and American Academy of Family Physicians.

19
■ ■ ■

Making Your Practice Palatable for Your Patients:
Cultural Competency

BARBARA P. YAWN

ANGELINE BUSHY

with

KATHY DUBBELS

PELAGE "MIKE" SNESRUD

CAROLE E. HILL

Introduction

Compared with urban centers, rural areas of the United States have a higher proportion of racial, ethnic, religious, and cultural minorities (Bushy, 1992). Many of these groups experience high levels of poverty, limited educational opportunities, and have little access to other people of similar ethnic backgrounds. This demographic trend, coupled with the fact that many rural counties do not have sufficient numbers of health care providers, can lead to severe restrictions on accessible health care (Lumsdon, 1993).

Deciding to establish a practice in a rural or underserved area is laudable. However, that alone may not be sufficient to assure that the residents of the rural area receive health care. Availability is not the same as accessibility. To be accessible the care must be desirable and familiar to the people you want to treat. What people find desirable or even acceptable is often based on their ethnic and cultural backgrounds. Cultural barriers to health care are not new. But the results of those barriers have become more obvious as we find the health outcomes of many groups to be less desirable than those of the urban middle-class Caucasian population.

This chapter will suggest ways to assess potential cultural barriers to the care you give. The process toward the provision of culturally competent or acceptable care begins with awareness followed by skills development and action. In addition to general principles, three specific overviews of non-Caucasian cultures will be presented.

Awareness of the Role of Culture

As with most problems the first step in resolution of cultural barriers to health care is the recognition of their roles in preventing people from seeking care and following treatment plans. Little is known about the health beliefs of many ethnic groups living across the 50 states. Their lifestyle behaviors may seem foreign to professionals who come to the rural regions to serve them. Even Anglo-Americans in rural areas may have beliefs and lifestyles that appear very unusual to their Anglo-American urban trained providers.

For example, as a lifelong resident of suburban middle America, I (Barbara Yawn) anticipated little difficulty in adjusting to life in rural Minnesota. As the first woman physician and family physician in a community of 10,000 people served by a multi-specialty group, I anticipated a few glitches—mainly from my partner colleagues. However, it did not take long to realize that I was an outsider, not because I was a woman professional but because I had no ancestors in this 100-year-old community and no farm blood in my veins. But with a genuine show of interest and enthusiasm for my new community I was accepted as an "educable" outsider.

In the town in which I practiced, everything stops on Wednesday evening—that is church night. You do not ask a farmer to return for a checkup during planting or harvesting (April to July and September to December). Giving advice is fine but you had better follow it at all times yourself because you can't go anywhere that someone doesn't recognize you. Joining a church is expected, as is a generous donation to the YMCA and the church. Your opinion is important but is more useful if confirmed by an older physician who has been around a few years (usually 20 or more).

A garden that is well tended, highly visible, and has some vegetable unusual for the region (like okra in Minnesota) is a plus. Admitting to a dislike of fresh corn is unwise, and you should never tell anyone what you do with all the zucchini you are given by patients and friends. Sunday afternoons should include a short drive in the country so you can comment on the progress of the crops, and be sure to listen to the weather report even if you don't have time to experience it. Always attend the community's one big annual festival and the county fair.

How do you acquire this knowledge? Although you can just jump right into the community, it is unlikely you will learn all the important facts before making some major blunders. The first step in learning to accommodate your new (or current) community's cultural background is to understand your own cultural background and how it affects what you think and do. Although there are many ways of looking at your own circles of culture, all assessments ask similar questions (Booth, 1992):

- How do you identify yourself in term of race, ethnic group, and socioeconomic class?
- What has it meant to be part of that group?
- Describe the customs or traditions in your family of origin that expressed your heritage. What special foods, gifts, songs, and ceremonies were related to events such as birth, puberty, starting school, graduation, marriage, divorce, and death?
- How were feelings like love and affection expressed in your family?
- How were feelings like anger and sadness expressed?
- What were the most valued and respected personal traits?
- What was the role of women in your family and culture?
- What was the role of men?
- How were decisions made?
- What role did fate play in a person's life?
- How was time defined and valued?
- What was your first experience with feeling different?

Answering these questions for ourselves and the members of our community can help physicians understand their own expectations of people when they are ill and compare them to the expectations of our patients. Some of these community expectations will become obvious as you work in the community. However, it is unlikely that you will learn about the groups that are not in the mainstream of your rural area unless you specifically seek them out.

The process of becoming more culturally competent involves moving from general awareness to a more sophisticated understanding of individuals coming from a different set of cultural circles. A first step is to learn about the history, geography, language, music, and customs of a defined group of people. Recreational reading can include biographies and fiction written by members of specific cultures. Social structures such as religion, politics, economics, law, technology, kinship, or education are taken into consideration to assess holistically how those environmental factors influence the group's health. Also of interest are the community's historical roots, its natural resources, food preferences, language, art forms, folktales, myths, symbols, and rituals. Increasingly there are plays and movies presented from a specific group's point of view. Such activities can provide background and a better sense of context when interacting with members of that group. It will not tell you everything about any specific member of that group. Still, this increased awareness of culturally driven behavior can explain puzzling or annoying differences in regards to time, authority, conflict, gender differences, and the role of the individual.

Individuals vary in the extent to which they exhibit their geopolitical and racial cultures. For immigrants and refugees, the length of time they have been in the country makes a difference. Language barriers, both spoken and written, make communication and acculturation into the majority culture more difficult. Generational differences affect the speed of acculturation with the younger generations acculturating faster. Economic status has also been demonstrated to be a factor, with the poor acting more "ethnic" (Booth, 1992).

We must not forget that the health care profession has its own "culture" that influences interactions between professionals, including the hierarchy of physicians, nurses, and technicians, and the relationship between professional and patient. People at the top of the hierarchy work in a culture defined by power and authority.

The power of the medical culture makes it hard for people to ask questions unless given specific permission. Therefore, those seeking care often do not seek clarification. Care providers often overestimate both what patients already know or understand and the clarity and appropriateness of their own explanations (Bushy, 1992). Taking time to have the patient explain the prescribed treatment plan, including how to take any medicine, can go a long way in improving communication. Even greater cultural competency is demonstrated by asking the person's point of view and collaborating rather than imposing a treatment plan. Although this takes more time in the beginning it can prevent many follow-up phone calls and visits due to uncompleted treatment programs.

When Cultural Sensitivity Is Mandatory for Success

Sometimes cultural sensitivity is helpful but not mandatory. At other times lack of cultural awareness will doom a program to failure. For instance, when considering the addition of a family planning clinic to a predominantly Mexican American county, questions to be considered must include:

- What is the meaning of pregnancy to the community?
- What is (are) the community's predominate religious denomination(s) and their theological stances regarding birth control, family planning, and pregnancy?
- What are their beliefs, values, and perceptions about public support for family planning clinics?
- What is the local fertility rate? Maternal-infant mortality rate? Adolescent pregnancy rate?
- How is an unplanned pregnancy viewed by the "typical" family; for example, a burden, blessing, or fulfilling assigned gender roles?
- How are male and female gender roles defined?
- What, if any, reproductive health concepts are included in local schools' health curricula? Who is responsible for teaching these courses? What is the instructor's background?
- What are the utilization patterns for reproductive services, particularly prenatal care providers?

- What are the perceived barriers to the use of existing family planning services, public health clinics, physicians, and alternative care providers?

Resources for
Gathering Cultural Information

Not all information needs to be gathered from the community itself. Recreational literature, including magazines such as *National Geographic* and *Newsweek,* plays, and television programs have already been mentioned as resources. A literature review is also an important step to determine what has or has not been written about your community's ethnic group and their acceptance of new programs.

For instance, a small hospital in a rural county is interested in contracting with the Indian Health Service to provide an alcohol treatment program for Native American people, specifically members of the Sioux tribe. The proposed program will integrate endogenous native healing practices with contemporary interventions for chemical dependency. Literature citations of probable interest to the program planners include descriptions and evaluations of similar programs for Native American tribes in other geographical areas, cultural reports on Plains Indians, descriptions of programs that integrate traditional and contemporary healing practices for other ethnic and cultural groups, and evaluation reports on innovative models of rural chemical dependency treatment programs. A review of the literature informs program planners, administrators, and clinicians so they can build on the experiences of others and, hopefully, avoid some of the same pitfalls.

Another method of obtaining information is to develop a group of key informants. For instance, a representative group of key informants for completing a needs assessment to implement an emergency clinic in a rural county should include interviews with formal and informal leaders from various towns in the county. Formal leaders include, among others, chief(s) of the fire and police department(s), a mortician who also provides ambulance services, the county's physicians, county commissioners, and the hospital's administrator and director of nursing. Even though formal leaders' viewpoints are important, informal leaders may be more in tune with the grassroots perspective regarding emergency services.

Examples of informal leaders who could serve as key informants include: a lay healer who also practices midwifery; a highly regarded woman who has a leading role in the homemakers' club; an elderly retired rancher identified as the local historian and the only surviving relative of the town's founder; chairpersons for the local chapters of Farm Bureau, Farmers Union, and Cow Bells; and high school athletic coaches (Rose, 1990).

Starting a New Practice

If you are planning to start a new practice or to join an existing one in any rural area, a pre-visit to the community offers an opportunity to obtain background data. It allows you to observe the local lifestyle and gives the community a chance to observe you. Looking for a house or an apartment to rent or buy is an opportunity to move about without appearing to be intrusive. Ask for a realtor who has been in the community for many years. As the new professional in town you will likely rate the senior partner in the agency and the senior banker. Both can provide a wealth of information. Listen to locally produced radio talk shows, because those programs usually reflect current community concerns. Read the community's newspaper.

A close-knit community has a way of protecting its interests, responding to outsiders, and testing strangers (Leininger, 1985; Turner, 1991). Health providers are viewed as "professional strangers" by a group until proven otherwise. For rural populations, the notion of insider versus outsider is often cited as a factor that can affect their acceptability of care even when services are physically accessible and available (Weinert & Long, 1991). Consequently, you must first gain entrance, then establish rapport with the community of interest.

How do you become accepted by a community or institution, particularly when outsiders are viewed with suspicion? The health professional may find it useful to view the community metaphorically as a theater having a front and back stage (Leininger, 1985). Being aware that each stage yields a particular kind of information can reduce the feelings of frustration when learning about an unfamiliar community.

The information revealed by the community's front stage generally consists of superficial, controlled, protected, and false responses. The actors (community members such as the realtor or banker) often display protective behaviors such as testing the provider's motives, disguising or hiding reality by offering misinformation, and demonstrating ambivalence about revealing truths to a stranger. Every rural community in the midwest has a "church on every corner." Few community members will point out the bar or "supper club" that occupies the opposite corner.

Some outsiders are tested more than others; the motives for this behavior are beyond the scope of this chapter. Strangers can, however, become friends. When feelings of trust, acceptance, and respect replace fear and distrust, the health professional is in a position to progress from front to back stage (Johnson, 1990).

As you progress, the information that is revealed has greater depth because the actors are more willing to share intimate secrets and treasured information (Spradley, 1980). The quantity and quality of back stage data tend to be rich and meaningful compared with the ambiguous and superficial information obtained at the front stage.

When You Need
the Information Yesterday

Although it is not possible to discuss all the ethnic groups found in rural America, the following sections will provide some basic information on three specific groups: a Southeast Asian group (the Hmongs), Native Americans or American Indian people, and African American people in the deep South. The sections are written by health professionals who have spent years studying and caring for the groups they describe.

Southeast Asians

KATHY DUBBELS

Southeast Asian people have come to the United States in several waves. The original groups were brought out as the United States withdrew from Vietnam. Others came as political refugees over the next several years. In the past 5 to 10 years many of the arriving refugees have lived in refugee camps for several years. The original refugees included many people who had held positions of wealth and prestige. Later refugees were often forced to spend many years in crowded camps and had little time and opportunity for education. The cultural diversity of the Southeast Asian groups is as great as the cultural diversity of the people of Europe. They do not speak the same language. Some, such as the Hmong, have never had a written language. Despite these differences some general rules of social structure and expectations of health care do exist.

Most Southeast Asians consider the physician a helper whose duty is to serve patients. Questions like "Why are you here?" can be interpreted to mean the doctor does not care. It is better to be less demanding and ask, "How can I help you?" or "What has happened that makes you come today?" When patients come in for care, they expect to receive something tangible from the doctor. Many families do not understand how to buy and use over-the-counter medications. Providing samples of aspirin or acetaminophen is important. They do understand the system of prescriptions and are pleased to prepare a home remedy such as lemon, hot water, and honey for a cough if it is written out on a prescription pad. Physicians should listen first; it is acceptable to check to make sure you understand, but then always give something tangible as part of the treatment.

Families initially may be resistant to Western technology and hospitalization. For instance, many believe that obstetrical ultrasound will harm the baby. In some instances this fear can be traced to the experience of having a family member who miscarried after an ultrasound examination—not unusual because ultrasound tests are often done to assess obstetrical problems. Families need more teaching about all procedures, what they are and why they are being done. Patients need time to process that information, to go back and talk about it with their families. Providers need to be more patient and to refrain from reacting negatively to the patient's need for more time.

The hospital environment is frightening and very unfamiliar to most Southeast Asian people. They fear that they will be harmed, and they may not understand why things are being done. Southeast Asians believe that ill people need special diets and not those provided by most hospitals. Families may prefer to bring food for the hospitalized patient, and it may be difficult to reach an agreement on special dietary requirements. For example, it is important for Hmong women to eat a special diet after childbirth. They drink hot water and eat chicken and rice specially prepared by relatives. Many Hmong women go hungry in the hospital because they do not have the foods consistent with their beliefs.

Most Southeast Asian cultures consider the man of the family to be the appropriate public spokesperson. This may mean that the wife will not bring herself or the children to the physician without being accompanied by her husband or her husband's mother. It is best to address the husband first and after establishing some level of comfort you can ask if it is acceptable to communicate directly with the wife.

Pregnancy and childbirth for Southeast Asian people involve many rituals and beliefs that must be understood to provide adequate care to the pregnant woman. Below are a few of the Hmong beliefs that are most likely to be contradicted by an unsuspecting physician.

- Taking a daytime nap will cause a long, difficult labor and delivery.
- A baby born at 7 months has a better chance of survival than if born at 8 months.
- No baby clothes should be purchased before the baby is born. This is a bad omen.
- During pregnancy it is alright to eat what you like.
- A good age to bear a child is between 13 and 19 years.
- If you place an eel in a jar of alcohol and drink the alcohol, your labor and delivery will be easier.
- The character of the baby may be like the persons assisting with the delivery.
- Drinking alcohol (strong, 80% proof) with herbs postpartum increases bleeding, which in turn promotes well-being.
- If you say aloud how good and cute the baby is, the bad spirit will think so too and may take the child (the child will get sick or die).

Knowing such beliefs can make it possible to talk to a pregnant woman and her family without immediately contradicting their beliefs of many generations. Most will compromise if given help understanding the importance of including both traditional beliefs and modern medicine. For example, it is often possible to convince the woman to take the self-prescribed alcohol (both during pregnancy and postpartum) as one teaspoonful every 4 to 6 hours. This will decrease the alcohol from 12 ounces in one day to less than 2 ounces per day.

Traditions surrounding serious illness, puberty, and death are also very specific and involved. Finding an interpreter and advocate who can help you understand these traditions will make the experience of caring for Southeast Asian people exciting, challenging, and rewarding.

American Indians or Native American People

PELAGE "MIKE" SNESRUD

Each Native American nation or tribe has its own history and belief system regarding health, illness, and traditional treatment. However, there are some general beliefs and practices that underlie the more specific tribal ideals. One is the traditional belief that health reflects living in total harmony with nature. The traditional belief holds that there is a reason for every sickness or pain: a price is being paid, either for something in the past or something that will happen in the future. These cause and effect relationships create an eternal chain. To many Native American people the state of health is regarded not only as the absence of disease but also as a reward for "good behavior." Illness is a punishment for bad behavior. Understanding these beliefs as well as how the individual perceives his state of wellness will help the provider. All too often there is a conflict between what Native Americans perceive their illness to be and what physicians may diagnose.

The Native American person and the provider may have differing perceptions of time. Life for many Native American people is not governed by the clock but by the dictates of need. Native Americans frequently may be late for specific appointments.

Communication with Native American people can be enhanced by realizing the importance they place on nonverbal communications. Often the Native American person will be observing the provider and saying very little. The patient may expect the physician to deduce through instinct rather than by the extensive use of questions during history taking. In part, this derives from the belief that "direct quoting" is intrusive upon individual privacy. When examining a Native American with an obvious cough, the provider might use a declarative statement such as "You have a cough that keeps you awake at night," and then allow time for the client to respond to the statement.

If a person appears to be experiencing significant pain but denies it when asked directly, try a less direct approach. "If your aunt, who I understand lives with you, were here in this room right now and I had a chance to talk with her, what would she tell me about the kind of day you had yesterday?" This puts the client in a position where she is speaking on behalf of someone else. This enables the disclosure of a great deal of information without being threatened. Any approach that you can take to create a nonthreatening physical environment for the person is helpful also. For example, assume similar height levels, either both sitting or standing, and assume sideways positions rather than a face-to-face stance.

Open-ended questions can be very useful. The patient often makes an appointment to be seen for a contrived reason, because she does not want to tell the receptionist the real problem, which is entirely different. Therefore it is critically important for the provider to allow the client to set the tone and the reasons for the visit and then to develop the care plan jointly.

It is Native American practice to converse in a very low tone of voice. It is expected that the listener will pay attention and listen carefully in order to hear what is being said. It is considered impolite to say, "I beg your pardon" or "What did you say?" or to give any indication that the communication was not heard. Therefore an effort should be made to speak with patients in a quiet setting where they will be heard more easily.

Note taking is taboo. Native America history has been passed through generations by means of storytelling. Native Americans are sensitive about note taking when they are speaking. When one is taking a history or interviewing it is preferable to use memory skills rather than to record notes.

In any health care relationship with Native American people you are not working with just the individual. You are relating to the entire extended family. The family views it that way and they want to be part of the plan of care. If they are not brought into the discussion and planning, the follow-up will never be completed.

We have found and have been told by many clients that Native American people value human compassion, integrity, and honesty most of all. Native American people want to trust that when they have an appointment they will be seen promptly with minimal waiting time and that the provider who sees them will be able to give them as much time as is needed.

African Americans

CAROLE E. HILL

African Americans who live in the U.S. South are, in many ways, as heterogenous as the diverse populations that make up U.S. society. Many of the characteristics that sterotypically define African Americans can be found in many other cultural groups. However, their history and social standing in U.S. society have created distinctive cultural and social characteristics that are quite distinct from that of the majority of physicians. This is especially true in the rural U.S. South where an overwhelming majority of African Americans live in poverty and have poor health. Cultural competency in the medical setting requires an understanding of and a respect for diverse cultural and social experiences and the skills to interpret and communicate within the context of African American interactions, expectations, beliefs, and behaviors. It is important for treating African American clients to be aware of cultural and social processes as well as cultural context.

African Americans are acutely aware of differentials in social status when they enter clinical settings. They are also aware of the disparities that exist between the health status of blacks and whites. This awareness guides their expectations of physicians and or treatment outcomes. Airhihenbuwa (1992) reports that when African Americans give an affirmative answer to the question "Can someone get AIDS from donating blood?" they may be responding to their strong distrust of white health care providers rather than indicating their true knowledge of disease transmission. This answer may reflect a belief that they may intentionally be infected with the AIDS virus, a legacy of the syphilis experiments in Tuskegee.

Physicians need to be aware that when they are talking to an individual African American about a treatment plan, they are often negotiating with an extended family as well. African Americans value collective decision making rather than individual decision making. They often consult with family or household members before making an important decision. The needs and priorities of the family or household are an important part of decisions made about their continued utilization of health services and their ability and willingness to follow through with a proposed treatment. Often, decisions have to be made between purchasing crucial household items and purchasing medicines.

A frequent comment African Americans make about their interactions with physicians is that they (the physicians) talk down to clients and assume that clients do not know what's wrong with them. This perception often delays visits to physicians by African Americans. They have a higher tolerance for discomfort from symptoms and often ignore minor discomforts (Jackson, 1982). Physicians need to know that once African Americans have decided upon treatment, they have often already diagnosed their illnesses. Self-diagnosis is quite common and is based upon a set of symptoms that they interpret as indicative of specific illnesses. The narratives used to communicate these symptoms to physicians are frequently based on different assumptions and beliefs about the manifestations and causes of the illnesses, especially among lower income African Americans. This does not, however, mean that they do not have an understanding of medical knowledge. Their descriptions are simply expressed in different terminology. For example, "high" and "low" blood are considered illnesses and are often reported to physicians or other clinical personnel in the U.S. South. Though often translated as hypertension by physicians, African Americans believe that prescribed medicines help very little because hypertension does not have symptoms and "high blood" does.

Physicians need to evaluate the congruity between their scientific terminology and the terminology of their clients. This can only take place if enough time is spent with clients so the physicians can delineate their clients' symptoms. Simply asking questions based on standard medical categories will elicit misleading answers. Physicians may conclude that clients either do not have certain illnesses or that they do not understand the symptoms of illnesses. Physicians, in addition, need to pay attention to how they write directions for taking medicines. For example, directing a client to take a pill after every meal assumes that everyone eats three meals each day. Likewise, directing clients to take a pill four times a day assumes congruence with their own conceptions of time. These assumptions may be misleading and may result in an incorrect diagnosis or an inappropriate treatment plan that serves to reinforce African American skepticism of the health care system.

Religious beliefs are an important part of African American culture. They guide their responses to illnesses and to medical treatment. Most, if not all, illnesses are framed within a belief system that reflects African and Christian heritages. Physicians need to be aware that these beliefs are fundamental to their patients' lives and account for the causes they attribute to illness and the behaviors necessary to treat and heal illnesses.

A physician may need to ask questions within the framework of a client's "believed in" causation. For example, if a client believes that his or her condition has been caused by someone "working roots," the physicians needs to ask questions about his or her preferred treatment and negotiate how the two systems of treatment can accommodate one another. African Americans frequently use roots and herbs, over-the-counter medicines, and/or traditional healers to diagnose and treat illnesses. Frequently, the medical and self-care systems are combined, although clients are reluctant to discuss their use of alternative treatments with physicians.

Finally, an important aspect of African American health behaviors involves a strong belief in self-involvement and self-control in clinical encounters and treatment. Physicians need to involve their African American clients in developing a treatment plan that is appropriate to their social and cultural beliefs and experiences.

Summary

As with any clinical skill, providing culturally sensitive and acceptable medical care will require knowledge and practice. You can begin simply by expressing your desire to understand the patients' problems and needs from their perspective. The first step may be as easy as asking people of color how they refer to their own community: black or Afro-American; Asian, Hmong, or Laotian; American Indian or Native American. To enhance the process, several sources of culturally sensitive materials for physician and patient education are listed. Most are inexpensive and will save time, frustration, and concern over misunderstood actions, reactions, and interactions.

References

Airhihenbuwa, C. (1992). Health promotion and disease prevention strategies for African-Americans: A conceptual model. In R. Braithwaite & S. Taylor (Eds.), *Health issues in the black community* (pp. 267-280). San Francisco: Jossey-Bass.

Booth, T. (1992). Cultural competence. *Perinatal Connection, 3*(3), 1-17. (Available from Minnesota March of Dimes, 4940 Viking Drive, Edina, MN 55435)

Bushy, A. (1992). Research in rural nursing. *Journal of Nursing Administration, 22*(1), 50-56.

Jackson, J. J. (1982). Urban black Americans. In A. Harwood (Ed.), *Ethnicity and medical care* (pp. 37-129). Cambridge, MA: Harvard University Press.

Johnson, J. (1990). *Selecting ethnographic informants*. Newbury Park, CA: Sage.

Leininger, M. (Ed.). (1985). *Qualitative research methods in nursing*. New York: Grune & Stratton.

Lumsdon, K. (1993, February 5). Patient centered care. *Hospitals*, pp. 14-26.

Rose, D. (1990). *Living the ethnographic life*. Newbury Park, CA: Sage.

Spradley, J. (1980). *Participant observation*. New York: Holt, Rinehart & Winston.

Turner, T. A. (1991). Health promotion for rural black elderly: Community-based program development. In A. Bushy (Ed.), *Rural nursing-Vol I*. Newbury Park, CA: Sage.

Weinert, C. & Long, K. A. (1991). The theory and research base for rural nursing practice. In A. Bushy (Ed.), *Rural nursing-Vol. I*. Newbury Park, CA: Sage.

Recommended Reading

Agar, M. (1981). *The professional stranger: An informal ethnography*. New York: Academic Press.

Braithwaite, R., & Taylor, S. (Eds.). (1992). *Health issues in the black community*. San Francisco: Jossey-Bass.

Chatters, L. M. (1991). Physical health. In J. S. Jackson (Ed.), *Life in black America* (pp. 199-220). Newbury Park, CA: Sage.

Dressler, W. (1991). *Stress and adaptation in the context of culture: Depression in a southern black community*. Albany: SUNY Press.

Hartman, D. (Ed.). (1982). *New directions for methodology of social and behavioral sciences. Using observers to study behavior*. San Francisco: Jossey-Bass.

Hill, C. E. (1988). *Community health systems in the rural American south: Linking people and policy*. Boulder, CO: Westview.

Hill, C. E. (1992). Reproduction and transformation of health praxis and knowledge among southern blacks. In H. B. Gender & Y. Jones (Eds.), *African-Americans in the south: Issues of race, class, and gender* (pp. 34-59). Athens: University of Georgia Press.

Jones, W., & Mitchell, F. (Eds.). (1987). *Health care issues in black Americans: Politics, problems, and prospects.* Westport, CT: Greenwood Press.

Snow, L. (1974). Folk medical beliefs and their implications for care of patients. *Annals of Internal Medicine, 81,* 82-96.

Snow, L. (1976). High blood is not high blood pressure. *Urban Health, 6,* 54-55.

Resources

AAPHCO, Asian Health Services
310 8th Street
Suite 200
Oakland, CA 94607
(415) 465-3272
(Maternal and child health education materials in Asian languages)

Asian American Health Forum
116 New Montgomery Street
Suite 531
San Francisco, CA 94105
(415) 541-0866
(Health information materials, Asian health newsletter)

County of Los Angeles
Department of Health Services
313 North Figueroa Street
Los Angeles, CA 90012
(213) 974-7764
(Nutrition materials for Hispanics)

Native American Women's Health Education Resource Center
P.O. Box 572
Lake Andes, SD 57356
(605) 487-7072
(Health information materials)

Pedersen, P. (1988). *A handbook for developing multicultural awareness.* Chicago: American Association of Counseling and Development.

Simonson, R., & Walker, S. (1988). *Multicultural literacy: Opening the American mind.* Ellensburg, WA: Graywolf Press.

Texas WIC Program. Low cost videos on prenatal nutrition, breastfeeding, baby care and nutrition. Distributed by:

Metro Post
501 N. Highway 35
Austin, TX 78702
(512) 476-3876
(Information for Hispanics)

White, E. C. (Ed.). (1990). *Black women's health care book: Speaking for ourselves*. Seattle, WA: Seal Press.

20
■ ■ ■

Ethics Dilemmas in Rural Practice

ANGELINE BUSHY

J. RANDALL RAUH

Introduction

Ethics dilemmas are usually identified in well-publicized incidents in metropolitan medical research centers (Rosner, 1985; Thomasma, 1985). However, rural health care practitioners also must face similar situations. Dilemmas relating to removal of life support, advance directives, the right to life, the right to die, termination of pregnancy, do-not-resuscitate orders, futility of care, and allocation of scarce resources occur in rural as well as in urban institutions.

The purpose of this chapter is to demonstrate the reality of ethics conflicts for rural physicians; to provide an overview of four fundamental ethics principles that are important in ethics decision making; and to describe the complex dimensions of an ethics conflict and the need for interdisciplinary discussions to arrive at a "best" decision. The chapter concludes with the application of the ethics decision making process to an obstetrical case involving a physician in rural practice.

Ethics Conflicts in Rural Settings

Rural practitioners are not exempt from ethics conflicts! The accuracy of this statement is illustrated by the following three incidents, all of which occurred in communities with less than 5,000 residents (Bushy & Rauh, 1991).

1. Greg, a 25-year-old farmer, is found to be HIV positive. He is not surprised but insists that the physician not inform his wife of the lab results. The couple have been married for 8 years and have two preschool children. Greg's mandate is in direct conflict with his physician's belief regarding the right of a spouse to be informed when a patient has a positive HIV test.

2. Lucy, 92 years old, suffered a severe heart attack 9 months ago. Since then she has been comatose and fed through a gastric tube. Recently her family demanded that all tube feeding be discontinued in order to respect Lucy's verbal request that "When the time comes, let me die in peace." Contrarily, the personnel in the nursing home, as well as the community at large, perceive the family's request as tantamount to "starving Lucy to death."

3. Steve, 37 years old, was transferred from a VA Hospital in California to the local nursing home. He was born in the community but has not resided here for about 30 years. He has a diagnosis of advanced cancer of the pancreas, but the community "rumor mill" attributes his emaciated condition to advanced stages of AIDS. Based on those reports, several of the nursing home's personnel refused to provide care to him. The institution has no written policy regarding care for residents with infectious diseases such as AIDS.

These situations reinforce the idea that rural as well as urban physicians are confronted with difficult ethics situations. There is a consensus that rural-urban differences in ethics considerations do exist. For instance, rural residents are described as more family oriented, frequently having extended family members residing within the same community. This can facilitate or hinder family consensus. Rural residents tend to be more conservative and traditional in their beliefs and show greater reluctance to adopt innovations. These attitudes are part of the rural value system and can affect health care seeking behaviors as well as the use of biotechnology. Rural values must be considered in ethics discussions relevant to rural patients (Weinert & Long, 1991).

The Ethics Decision-Making Process

The first step in the decision making process (Table 20.1) is to identify your personal values regarding health, health care, and medical practice, and then to compare and contrast those with

Table 20.1 Overview of the Ethical Decision-Making Process

- Self-appraisal of personal values and beliefs
- Comparison of self-appraisal with professional code of ethics
- Determine congruence of self-appraisal, professional code of ethics with institutional mission
- Define the problem
- Identify the patient
- Identify treatment options
- Consider all real and potential environmental influences for each treatment option (e.g., advance directives; patient/family/community value systems)
- Assess benefits, risks, and outcomes of each option on patient/family society/providers using ethics principles
- Appraise consequences of each option
- Implement the most appropriate intervention

medicine's code of ethics. This self-appraisal means identifying congruencies and differences in values and beliefs. You are then in a position to evaluate how personal and professional values mesh with the mission of a particular health care institution. Next you decide if you are willing to practice within that particular setting. Such a self-appraisal better prepares any physician to address ethics conflicts that might be encountered in medical practice.

When a difficult situation occurs, you must determine if the problem really is an ethics conflict, a medical conflict, a legal conflict, or a combination of these. If it is an ethics problem, two major points must be clarified: Exactly who is the patient and what actions, treatments, or consequences are being considered. Who the patient is may not be as simple as it sounds as in the case of a mentally incompetent person, a child, a person with the diagnosis of Alzheimer's disease, or a sedated patient. Likewise, depending on the laws of a state, an ethics decision could be predetermined by advance directives such as a living will (May, 1975; Thomasma, 1985).

Next, you must ascertain the consequences of each option or medical intervention (Memel, 1987; Nelson, 1987). The analysis includes identifying outcomes that may result from each action or the lack of action. Ethicists generally concur that undoing treatment is more difficult than withholding initial treatment of a patient, such as inserting a feeding tube, or initiating intravenous therapy or mechanical ventilation. Therefore withholding treatment also should be considered as an alternative. Consider whether the outcomes of an intervention will serve to increase or decrease patient and family suffering, improve their quality of life, postpone the patient's death, or contribute to death. Physicians must always be sensitive to the patient's value system when considering an ethics conflict.

Because of the complexity of most ethics situations, one or two individuals are not in a position to anticipate the full ramifications. The courts have mandated that ethics decisions be made by those having medical expertise as opposed to resolving ethics decisions in the legal arena. However, legal ramifications infringe on many ethics decisions, and a practitioner always must consider the medicolegal consequences of any actions. The consequences to physicians of making ethics decisions can range from slight personal remorse, a malpractice suit, loss of professional license or, in some instances, incarceration. The far-reaching ramifications of ethics conflicts support the need for intra- and interdisciplinary discussions. An ethics committee, if available, is an appropriate forum for ethics debates. Physicians in rural practice have a responsibility to be informed and actively represented in those discussions.

Ethics Decision Making:
A Case Analysis

To demonstrate the reality of an ethics conflict occurring in a rural setting, an obstetrical case is presented. The situation encompasses medical, social, and economic dimensions pertinent to rural environments. The ethics principles of autonomy, beneficence, utility, and justice are employed to analyze the case. The medical approaches in this case may differ; and we concede that this discussion is by no means a final stance for the case, and that we do not address all of the potential legal consequences. The intent is to demonstrate the need for in-depth discussion regarding these kinds of situations, even in small, rural institutions (Bushy & Rauh, 1991).

Case Presentation

Joan is 22 weeks pregnant when she first visits Dr. Smith, the only obstetrician within a 150-mile radius. Joan and her husband Mike have delayed visiting the doctor because of financial problems. Since the beginning of this pregnancy she has had intermittent episodes of vaginal bleeding and now seeks medical care because of heavy bleeding. Upon examination the doctor informs Joan that she has an incompetent cervix; thus, delivery of a preterm fetus is highly probable.

Joan's obstetric and social history indicate she has had six pregnancies, four of which ended in spontaneous miscarriages. Two pregnancies resulted in live births, one being the premature delivery of a son at 7 months. Because of his prematurity, 4-year-old Tommy is neurologically impaired, mentally retarded, and prone to pulmonary problems. His condition has incurred additional expenses for medication, physician visits, and rehabilitation. He will continue to require special education and extensive physical therapy. The child's condition has been a burden both emotionally and financially, but the parents have assumed full responsibility for his care. They repeatedly state that Tommy has brought many joys to their family. Another of Joan's pregnancies resulted in the term delivery of a son John, now 8 months old and developmentally normal.

Mike and Joan "were born and raised Catholic" in this midwest town. Most of their extended family live here and provide support to the couple. Despite the depressed economy, Mike is employed as a farm laborer and Joan has been able to remain home with the children. The couple has health insurance that includes a prohibitive deductible cost, does not include coverage for emergency transfer, or reimburse for neonatal intensive care.

Considering Joan's status, the obstetrician outlines treatment options to the couple.

1. Have Joan continue with her usual activities of daily living and not initiate any medical intervention, that is, let nature take its course.
2. Have Joan begin medication for the bleeding and restrict her to bed rest. With two small children this probably is not realistic so she may need to be hospitalized.
3. Have the obstetrician perform a minor surgical procedure (cerclage) to maintain the uterine cervix in a closed position with sutures until closer to Joan's due date.

The couple expresses understanding of the urgency of the situation and consent to the minor surgical procedure, which is performed. Joan returns home, but 2 weeks later she is again admitted to the hospital for premature labor and placed on medication in an attempt to stop the contractions. Despite these interventions her contractions and bleeding persist, and delivery seems imminent.

The doctor informs the couple that if the fetus is to have any chance for survival Joan can no longer be treated at this small hospital. The risks are outlined: at 25 weeks gestation the fetus has only a 10% survival rate even in a highly specialized neonatal care unit located 800 miles away. If the newborn survives, there is at least a 50% chance that it will have some type of long-term disability.

Based on the estimated risk factors two options emerge. The first is to remove the cervical sutures and discontinue all medications. This option will probably result in delivery of an immature fetus in the local hospital. But this option is complicated by the fact that the only pediatrician on the medical staff is out of town. During this time a general practitioner with limited neonatal experience is on call for pediatric patients. Even with the use of all of the available resources in the small hospital, it is highly likely that the newborn would probably die before being transferred to the tertiary medical center.

The second option is to transfer Joan to the tertiary medical center before delivery so that neonatal intensive care can be instituted promptly after birth. This requires chartering emergency air transportation and, considering the limited insurance benefits, imposes a financial burden on the couple. The estimated total cost for this care is between $100,000 and $200,000. A conflict between the couple and the obstetrician emerges.

On the one hand, the couple is adamant about having Dr. Smith deliver Joan in the local hospital. Their decision is based on the reality that they cannot absorb the financial and emotional costs of Joan delivering the baby in the distant medical center. Contrarily, the obstetrician perceives the parents' request to be tantamount to a late second trimester abortion. His position is based on the probable consequence of removing the cervical sutures without the immediate availability neonatal intensive care services. His reluctance is reinforced by the facts that this is a Catholic hospital, that there are conflicting legal opinions for similar cases, and that there is a possibility of being involved in litigation over the matter.

Table 20.2 Ethics Principles

ETHICAL NORM

> A statement (principle) that actions of a certain type ought (or ought not) to be done.

AUTONOMY

> Respect for individuals who act autonomously (not others) to make decisions that affect their lives.

PATERNALISM

> Limiting an individual's liberty when his or her actions might result in harm, or fail to produce an important benefit.

BENEFICENCE

> Acts of kindness; an obligation of doing or promoting good for another; "Do no harm"; maximize possible benefits and minimize possible harm.

UTILITY

> The greatest good/happiness for the greatest number.

JUSTICE

> Equals should be treated equally. Those who are unequal should be treated differently according to their differences.

Discussion

Situational ethics is defined as a case-by-case approach to resolving ethics situations. Generally speaking, this approach denies the usefulness of ethics principles and can be risky, both ethically and legally. Instead, it is wiser to use a logical approach to resolve a situation, using ethics norms and fundamental principles (Table 20.2) to guide decision making (Gaffney, 1979; Schneiderman, 1993). Any number of social, economic, legal, and ethics questions surround Joan's case—all of which affect the selection of a "best" intervention. When one considers all of the dimensions, it quickly becomes evident that a single individual is not in a position to ascertain the full implications of each option (Lagerlof, 1988).

Questions that must be resolved in Joan's case include: Who is the patient, that is, the mother, the pregnant family (mother, father, and living children), or the fetus? How is abortion defined, by whom, and whose definition carries the greatest weight, that is, the mother, the pregnant family, the physician, or the state? What weight does the decision of the marital bond carry in the treatment choice for the pregnant wife? How does society ascertain the short- and long-term effects of each option on the mother, the family, the physician, the rural community, and society? In relation to the rural setting, how do you evaluate the financial and social costs of transporting Joan to a distant medical center in order to provide intensive care for her newborn?

The principles of autonomy, beneficence, utility, and justice will be used to argue Joan's case. Depending upon the principle that is used, the interventions chosen for Joan may differ and in some cases may be markedly different.

Autonomy

The principle of autonomy infers respect for individuals in that they are able to act autonomously. It infers that each person (not others) can make decisions that affect his or her life. Autonomy directs that a patient's values are of the highest priority and should guide a physician's treatment regimen. Inherent in autonomy is the concept of informed consent, that is, the right of competent adults to accept or refuse medical treatment on the basis of full information from the health care provider. To assure autonomy of a mentally incompetent person a responsible individual (proxy) must make decisions for him or her (Freel, 1985).

Self-determination takes precedence over the values of medicine. For example, when a mentally competent pregnant woman requests a medical intervention or procedure that has medical benefit, the physician must comply with her requests. Thus, Dr. Smith is obligated to provide all of the "available treatment" within the rural hospital to Joan and her fetus. Autonomy also allows for the general practitioner who practices in town to care for the high-risk infant in the absence of the pediatrician.

In Joan's case the fetus can also be viewed as a patient, but an incompetent one. If a provider uses this approach, it requires that the parents, acting as a proxy, must make a quality-of-life decision for their unborn child. Their decision is based on the assumption that their child has a high risk of being disabled because of prematurity.

Identifying the patient in this case is complex. Whose autonomy takes precedence—Joan's? The fetus's? The parents', who are a proxy for the fetus versus their two living children? The physician's? The hospital's? The state's? Society's? What impact does Joan's signed surgical consent to maintain her pregnancy have on the autonomy of her fetus? On a broader perspective, can society require a pregnant woman to undergo treatment against her will (Ashley & Rourke, 1982; Bayley, 1982)?

The situation becomes even more obscure with some state legislation regarding the legal rights of a fetus. These laws may create an atmosphere where pregnant women will be reluctant to acknowledge a pregnancy; or they may refuse to obtain prenatal care because of the threat of losing custody of the child or facing criminal prosecution. Specifically, what impact will this trend have on medical practice and health care delivery in medically underserved communities?

In Joan's case, questions generated by the principle of autonomy can be summarized as a threefold conflict:

- between a physician and a patient's right to autonomy
- between the physician's and patient's rights to privacy and the state's interests (legal issues)
- between the doctor-patient relationship and national standards of medical practice

For situations involving only one individual, the principle of autonomy may take precedence. In cases having two or more patients, such as a pregnant woman, this principle may be inappropriate. Considering the numerous individuals involved in Joan's situation, the principle of autonomy may not be practical because everyone's autonomy cannot be respected and fulfilled.

Beneficence

The principle of beneficence is doing or promoting good for another; it can conflict with the principle of autonomy. It can imply that a physician knows what is in the best interest of the patient (paternalism). With beneficence a medical regimen can be implemented on the basis of a doctor's expertise, regardless of a patient's wishes. Paternalism is used to justify limiting an individual's liberty when his or her actions might result in harm, or might fail to produce an important benefit to that person. Other examples of this concept are determining whether or not to tell a patient the truth about a poor medical prognosis, restraining someone who is believed to be suicidal, or committing someone into an institution of any kind (Freel, 1985).

An inferred concept within beneficence is nonmaleficence, which means to avoid intending, causing, permitting, or imposing harm or risk of harm to any person. It is conceivable that allowing a person to suffer may be more harmful than the death of a loved one. Family suffering often results from the imposed social, economic, and psychosocial circumstances of prolonged illness.

Specifically, if Joan is identified as the patient, one can argue that having a child who is impaired may cause extreme financial and emotional stress on the family. If the physician's primary intent is to do no harm and to relieve pain and suffering, beneficence would allow for Joan to have the baby in the small hospital. Logically, beneficence can support the notion that at times abortion may be in the mother's and family's best interest. Is this applicable to Joan's case?

If the fetus is identified as the patient, beneficence requires that intensive, sophisticated medical interventions be provided to the premature newborn. Extraordinary measures are required even though neonatal intensive care services are located 800 miles away, and despite the excessive costs to the family, third-party payers, and the rural town's social service coffers. The situation is further complicated when one considers the comparatively few people who have resources to contribute, as is the case in frontier regions of the United States. Depending upon whether the focus is on Joan or her fetus, the principle of beneficence could either support or refute having the delivery in the local hospital.

Utility

The principle of utility is entirely pragmatic and supports the notion of the greatest good or happiness for the greatest number. It infers balancing the good that is possible to do with the harm that might result from doing, or not doing, the deed (Ashley & Rourke, 1982). To assist in allocating scarce resources, ethicists have developed a hierarchical structure to prioritize benefits and resources. Among others, psychological happiness has the highest priority, followed by financial happiness.

Prioritizing and allocating scarce resources has serious implications for economically depressed rural communities. Despite the intent of "fairness," prioritizing raises additional questions. For example, should one consider short-term or long-term happiness? Whose happiness? Who determines the greatest numbers and how does one measure the nebulous concept of "happiness"? If psychological happiness is prioritized over financial happiness, how do the costs and benefits compare for a rural family of five versus society? Obviously, if numbers are of paramount consideration, the family loses and society becomes the only priority. Particular concerns also emerge regarding the proper use of medical resources in less populated and economically deprived geographic regions.

Based on the experiences of other families confronting similar obstetrical circumstances, one can only speculate as to the long- and short-term psychological and financial costs imposed on Joan's family. Yet, despite the risks of permanent disability of the baby, how does one ascertain what this child might contribute over a lifetime to the family and society? Obviously, there are quality-of-life issues at stake for all involved, but whose definition takes precedence?

If the principle of utility focuses on the physician, one can speculate that he might have some degree of short-term happiness secondary to facilitating Joan's and Mike's happiness. Then again, there may be inherent guilt, stress, grief, and unhappiness incurred by his treatment. Moreover, depending upon how abortion is defined, the consequences of his action could result in a legal conviction or revocation of a medical license. Much like the logic related to autonomy and beneficence, the principle of utility can support either Joan's or Dr. Smith's position as to where the baby should be delivered (Gaffney, 1979).

Justice

The principle of justice implies that equals should be treated equally and that those who are unequal should be treated differently according to their differences. Equal treatment does not necessarily mean identical treatment. Instead, equality refers to contributions that promote relative, similar goodness in the life of those not considered to be equal. This could mean providing greater (than equal) opportunity or service to the less fortunate to enable them to achieve benefits comparable to those of more fortunate counterparts. In regard to allocation of resources, distributive justice can be according to equal shares or preferential treatment based on need, merit, or societal contribution. This approach obviously raises questions related to universal access to health care, particularly in medically underserved rural regions.

How could the principle of justice affect rural communities, considering the prevailing poverty and the high incidence of vulnerable populations having fewer formal social services available to them? Should rural populations be expected to relinquish some degree of access to health care in lieu of a preferred lifestyle? If so, how much, and who determines the ratio between access to care versus a preferred lifestyle? Contemporary philosophers are viewing the principle of justice as preferential consideration for those who are most prone to unjust treatment, inferring the least advantaged should receive the most resources. Societal benevolence of this magnitude raises a more practical concern: Who pays?

In Joan's case we must ask who is most disadvantaged or most prone to unjust treatment? Logically, one can conclude that it may be Joan, the family, or the unborn fetus. Joan might be perceived as the most disadvantaged when one considers her role of primary caretaker of three preschool children, one of whom is, and another who might be, physically, emotionally, or mentally challenged. The family could be perceived as the most disadvantaged because of the medical hardships imposed by a second disabled child. Or, the fetus could be perceived as most disadvantaged because of its immaturity. Depending upon who is identified as least fortunate in Joan's case, interdisciplinary discussion is needed to assess the psychological pain, financial distress, and social problems imposed on others (Thomasma, 1985).

On a more global perspective some might identify society as being the most disadvantaged because of the costs incurred by adding another human being to an overextended health care system on an over-populated planet. This stance stems from environmental issues, limited resources, economic inequities (poverty), and excessive taxation. Hence, the principle of utility and preferential treatment is perceived as a Christian-utopian ideal. Because of the numerous individuals involved, justice might not be an appropriate rationale for Joan's case (Ashley & Rourke, 1982).

Outcome

The obstetrician asked for a consultation with the other four physicians at the hospital, the priest, the minister on chaplaincy call for the hospital, and the hospital administrator. The majority of the group gave greater weight to the principal of autonomy, and concluded that the woman had the right to demand local treatment. The obstetrician was not comfortable with this decision, and withdrew as the treating physician. He did agree to be available to help with any obstetrical emergencies.

The new attending physician found that Joan's labor had continued to progress, and she delivered 2 hours later. The gestational age of the infant was indeed 23-25 weeks. The baby had a few gasping respirations and a pulse of 70. Resuscitative measures including intubation, ventilation by Ambu bag, umbilical venous catheterization, and cardiac massage were undertaken, but the infant died within 1 hour.

Recommendations

Joan's case demonstrates that ethics conflicts are not clear-cut situations that have a black or white solution—there are many shades of gray. In order to consider all the dimensions of an ethics conflict rural physicians must be educated about ethics theory and terminology. They also must be aware of resources such as ethics committees or ethicists who can be consulted should an ethics event present in geographically and professionally isolated rural practice settings. It is important to initiate interdisciplinary ethics discussions in rural health care institutions before a problem occurs. These discussions can do much to promote ethics awareness in an institution while educating professionals about the ethics decision making process. A case analysis such as the discussion of Joan's case is an effective strategy for creating ethics awareness, educating staff on the topic of ethics, and facilitating interdisciplinary discussions that establish clinical relevance to the ethics decision making process (Aroskar, 1984; Cranford, Hester, & Ashley, 1985; Niemira, Orr, & Culver, 1989; Rosner, 1985).

The following points are standards for group work that will facilitate the function of any ethics group or committee (Ashton, 1993).

- **All opinions have equal status.** Often it is the most unusual and unconventional idea that is the most useful and prudent in developing collective wisdom.
- **Group members must listen to the satisfaction of the sender of the message.** It is absolutely essential to listen to the speaker and hear his or her intent. Respect each other as well as the speaker. Listen to learn; listen nondefensively; listen without discount. Do not prepare your response while a speaker is speaking. Do not respond or interrupt until another has finished speaking. Hear the person out to the end of the comment.
- **Group members respect the confidentiality of the group.**
- **Group members address issues and concerns directly with those involved.** No gossip; use direct, specific disagreement and avoid passive-aggressive behaviors at later times within the group or outside of the group setting.
- **Once we reach consensus, we will speak with "one voice" about the issue.** Avoid "behind the back" or "under the table" comments; make no undermining or second guessing comments to the public about the group's decision.
- **Aim for win-win situations; use negotiation rather than confrontational approaches.** People generally are more satisfied receiving part of a request rather than none at all so long as the decision is perceived as "fair."

Summary

Ethics conflicts take a tremendous toll on all involved. The burden stems from the high degree of uncertainty associated with various biomedical options, as well as conflicting value systems that exist among families, health professionals, state statutes, and religious doctrine. Education of health professionals and the public regarding the importance of advance directives, making informed decisions, and establishing realistic expectations from a medical intervention are first steps in avoiding ethics conflicts. Should conflicts occur, health professionals need to be comfortable with the interdisciplinary nature of addressing ethics situations.

References

Aroskar, M. (1984). Considerations in establishing an ethics committee. *Association of Operating Room Nurses Journal, 40,* 88-92.

Ashley, B., & Rourke, K. (1982). *Health care ethics: A theological analysis.* St. Louis: Catholic Healthcare Association.

Ashton, C. (1993, April). *Facilitating the group process.* Paper presented at the Annual Utah Organization of Nurse Executives, Salt Lake City.

Bayley, C. (1982, April 8). Institutional approach: Ethics committees and consuls. Presented at *Proceedings of the American Society of Law and Medicine,* Los Angeles, CA.

Bushy, A., & Rauh. J. (1991). Ethical dilemmas: Do they occur in rural practice? In A. Bushy (Ed.), *Rural nursing-Vol. 2,* (pp. 203-214). Newbury Park, CA: Sage.

Cranford, R., Hester, F., & Ashley, B. (1985). Institutional ethics committees: Issues of confidentiality and immunity. *Law Medical Health Care, 13,* 52-60.

Freel, M. (1985). Truth telling. In J. McClosky & H. Grace (Eds.), *Current issues in nursing.* Boston: Blackwell Scientific Publishers.

Gaffney, J. (1979). *Newness of life.* St. Louis: Paulist Press.

Lagerlof, J. (1988, January-February). Maternal fetal conflict. *California Nursing Review,* pp. 34-36.

May, W. (1985). The composition and function of ethics committees. *Journal of Medical Ethics, 1,* 23-29.

Memel, S. (1987). When do ethical issues become legal issues? *Health Executive, 2(5),* 46-49.

Nelson, S. (1987). Liability issues increasing ethics consultations. *Hospitals, 61(9),* 80-84.

Niemira, D., Orr, R., & Culver, C. (1989). Ethics committees in small hospitals. *Journal of Rural Health, 5(1),* 19-32.

Rosner, M. (1985). Hospital ethics committees: A review of their development. *Journal of the American Medical Association, 253(18),* 2693-2697.

Schneiderman, L. (1993). Futility in practice. *Archives of Internal Medicine, 153,* 437-441.

Thomasma, D. (1985). Hospital ethics committees and hospital policy. *Quarterly Review Bulletin, 11,* 204-209.

Weinert, C., & Long, K. (1991). The theory and research base for rural nursing practice. In A. Bushy (Ed.), *Rural nursing-Vol. I,* (pp. 21-38). Newbury Park, CA: Sage.

Recommended Reading

Gannon, T. M. (Ed.). (1987). *Catholic challenge to the American economy: Reflections on the U.S. Bishops Pastoral Letter on Catholic Social Teachings in the U.S. Economy.* New York: Macmillan.

21
■ ■ ■

Quality Assessment in Rural Practice

PETER G. HARPER

CHARLES E. McCOY

ANGELINE BUSHY

Introduction

The decade of the 1990s will be a time of reform for health care systems. Access, accountability, and affordability are the key foci of the necessary changes. This chapter deals with the accountability aspect of health system change. Accountability for costs and outcomes is the primary factor associated with quality. Outcomes accountability includes assessment of morbidity and mortality, and consumer and provider satisfaction. Cost accountability includes proof of efficacy and appropriate utilization of services and technology. Although these terms can be intimidating, they are part of the foundation of every practitioner's daily activities. We want to improve the health outcomes of our patients in a cost-conscious manner that provides satisfaction for our patients and professional satisfaction and rewards for ourselves.

Rural hospitals, physicians' offices, and emergency departments are now, or soon will be, faced with the same demands for accountability and cost outcomes data that large urban centers and health maintenance organizations have to address. In the rural setting the

AUTHORS' NOTE: Adapted by Barbara P. Yawn from *The Family Practice Guide to Quality Improvement* by P. G. Harper & C. E. McCoy (Eds.), 1992, Minneapolis: Minnesota Academy of Family Physicians. Copyright 1992 by Minnesota Academy of Family Physicians. Adapted by permission.

number of people served is smaller, but so is the availability of people and systems to collect and evaluate the relevant information. Not all rural facilities have computerized data systems, and most of those with computers use them only for billing and accounting rather than for clinical data applications. The numbers of people with specific diagnoses and procedures may be so small that meaningful statistical evaluation may be difficult. Support resources for data collection, analysis, and interpretation are often nonexistent in smaller communities. The need for clinical data collection and analysis can be met by grouping or networking of small hospitals and physicians, support from regional or state primary care research networks, and the development of some local expertise.

Measuring and assuring quality have been the purported goals of quality assurance activities in hospitals. Usually dictated by outside groups such as Medicare or the Joint Commission on Accreditation for Healthcare Organizations (JCAHO), these quality activities are often time-consuming and frustrating. Physicians recognize the intrinsic benefits of evaluation, improvement, and reassessment, and have persisted in looking for a method of quality assessment that meets their needs as well as those of regulating agencies. Continuous Quality Improvement (CQI) may be that system. The introduction of CQI will be discussed first in the context of the hospital and then transferred to the outpatient setting. Examples are provided to enhance understanding.

Hospital Quality Assessment

Monitoring and evaluation for quality improvement (QI) purposes can be a complex, time-consuming task for hospitals of all sizes; but this may be particularly problematic for small and rural hospitals. Historically, small rural hospitals have not fared as well as their urban counterparts in external accreditation surveys, especially by the JCAHO. That is not to say that small and rural hospitals do not have high-quality services. Rather, these facilities may use different approaches to providing services and measuring the quality of that care. *The Guide to Surveying Small and Rural Hospitals* (JCAHO, 1992) is an attempt to create sensitivity regarding the needs and strategies of these health care facilities.

In its 1990 quality assurance standards the JCAHO specifies a process by which the quality of care is monitored and evaluated. This process—which had been in effect for several years—involves identifying problems, assigning responsibility, requesting the responsible party to change, and then reassessing. This externally imposed process demands the identification of problems and forces practices to fit standards, rather than modifying standards to fit patient and facility characteristics and needs.

Alternatively, the CQI process suggests that health care quality can most effectively be improved by focusing on system failures, not by assigning fault. The steps of CQI are identification of key processes that affect patient care and outcomes, collection of data, defining the extent of problems in that process, and focusing on opportunities to improve the process.

The opportunities to improve care will be found by examining the systems and processes by which care is provided. These processes cross departmental and service lines, necessitating interdepartmental communication and coordination.

Thus to improve quality continuously, an entire organization from the governing body to the support services should be committed to a cooperative effort to improve care. Care will be improved not by focusing on outliers or "bad apples." Rather, care is improved by assessing and monitoring the complex series of activities that compose any key function in the hospital (Table 21.1). For example, the processes involved in medication use—prescribing, purchasing, ordering, preparing, dispensing, administering, and monitoring effects on patients—comprise intricate steps that are performed by physicians, nurses, pharmacists, and other staff. Improvements in this process will result from eliminating redundant steps, overly complex activities, and barriers to communication.

To carry out such quality improvement, meaningful data on how the system currently operates will be necessary. The usefulness of these data will depend on the development of valid performance measures, the application of reliable data collection techniques, appropriate statistical methods, and effective methods to disseminate the information to the proper audience. None of these steps can be accomplished by any single professional or support service group.

The concept of CQI incorporates the strengths of QI while broadening its scope, refining its approach to assessing and improving

Table 21.1 Outline of the JCAHO 10-Step Quality Improvement Process

1. Assign responsibility
   a. Involve organization leaders.
   b. Design and foster the approach to continuous improvement of quality.
   c. Set priorities for assessment and improvement.
2. Delineate the scope of care and service
   a. Identify key functions and/or identify the procedures, treatments, and other activities performed in the organization.
3. Identify important aspects of care and services
   a. Determine the key functions, treatments, processes, and other aspects of care/service that warrant ongoing monitoring.
   b. Establish priorities among the important aspects of the care/service chosen.
4. Identify indicators
   a. Identify teams to develop indicators for the important aspects of care service.
   b. Select the indicators.
5. Establish thresholds for evaluation
   a. Each team identifies thresholds for each indicator.
   b. Select the thresholds.
6. Collect and organize data
   a. Each team identifies data sources and data collection methods for the recommended indicators.
   b. The data collection methodology is designed, and those responsible for collecting, organizing, and applying thresholds are identified.
   c. Collect data
   d. Organize data so thresholds for evaluation can be applied.
   e. Collect data from other sources, including patient and staff surveys, comments, suggestion, and complaints.
7. Initiate evaluation
   a. Apply thresholds for evaluation to indicator data.
   b. Initiate evaluation of aspects of care/service if threshold is reached.
   c. Assess other feedback (e.g., staff suggestions, patient satisfaction survey results) that may contribute to priority setting for evaluation.
   d. Set other priorities for evaluation.
   e. Teams undertake intensive evaluation.
8. Take action to improve care and service
   a. Teams recommend and/or take actions (e.g., education, change policy procedure, individual counseling).
9. Assess the effectiveness of actions and maintain the gain
   a. Assess whether the care/service has improved.
   b. If not, further action is determined.
   c. (a) and (b) are repeated until improvement is achieved and maintained.
   d. Monitoring is maintained and priorities for monitoring and the indicators are periodically reassessed.
10. Communicate results to relevant individuals and groups
    a. Teams forward conclusions, actions, and results to leaders and to relevant individuals, committees, departments, and services.
    b. Disseminate information as necessary.
    c. Leaders and others receive and disseminate comments, reactions, and information from involved individuals and groups.

care, and dispensing with the negative connotations often associated with QI. Ultimately, the coordinated, comprehensive, systematic efforts associated with CQI will result in a continuous cycle of assessment and improvement.

Most physicians have participated in hospital-based QI or even CQI activities. But in today's changing health care systems, quality assessment must extend from the inpatient setting into the ambulatory practice. Many large clinics and HMOs have spent several years developing and refining CQI in outpatient clinics. The remainder of this chapter will focus on the implementation of quality improvement in small, rural outpatient practices.

Outpatient Quality Assessment

Whether in a large or small group the process of CQI must have the support of physicians, staff, and administration. Just as in the hospital, quality will be evaluated in the context of processes— patient flow, timely appointments, or follow-up of abnormal laboratory tests. These processes or systems involve every member of the group and cannot be assessed, evaluated, or improved without everyone's help.

Although CQI is best done by multidisciplinary work groups with a facilitator (not always a physician or administrator), the process still requires a leader or coleaders. Larger practices may appoint a QI committee that selects topics, appoints work groups, appropriates funds, and oversees the entire process. In a small group, separate committees are inappropriate; the entire staff can serve as the QI committee. The QI leader can be a physician, a nurse, a receptionist, or an administrator who feels comfortable assuming this responsibility and becoming the local expert on quality improvement techniques.

The CQI Process

The CQI process can be thought of as a loop (see Figure 21.1). To begin a CQI project you must identify a suitable topic or area to study. Extra care at this stage can make QI a straightforward and interesting process that leads to real improvement in patient care.

- Identify a topic or issue
- Assess the dimension of the issue
- Focus the study
- Develop criteria and set goals
- Assess care and report results
- Improve care
- Remeasure
- Report

Figure 21.1. The CQI Process

Most clinics can easily identify many areas that could be improved. Physician and staff suggestions, patient complaints, an occasional malpractice case, patient satisfaction surveys, and ongoing monitoring of deaths and incident reports will generate many topics. Good topics are common, important, correctable, and amenable to consensus.

Because only a few QI studies will be done each year, selecting common topics will affect a larger percentage of patients and practice procedures. You can identify your most common diagnoses from encounter or billing data analysis.

Example: Following a CME meeting, one of your partners reports that the latest recommendations for the care of people with diabetes include yearly retinal evaluations. Diabetes constitutes your ninth most common diagnosis. What are your current practices regarding eye care of these patients?

In the past there has been little to gain from studying topics with minor morbidity such as upper respiratory infections (URIs). But as cost and efficacy become more significant we should consider some topics in which morbidity is minor and physician care is of questionable benefit.

Example: URIs are the third most common diagnosis during the fall and winter months in a rural practice. Why are patients coming into the physicians' office for care? With appropriate patient education and triage could most of the patients with URI be self-treated?

The conditions you select for study should be correctable within the scope of CQI. Stick to topics that can be influenced by provider, staff, or systems adjustments.

Example: Cytobrushes can improve the chances of getting endocervical cells on a Pap test. Do providers currently routinely obtain endocervical cells on Pap tests? Provider education could increase cytobrush use in your practice if you are not meeting your goals.

The best QI topics are those in which there is agreement regarding the process of care at the national, state, and local levels. In many areas of medicine there is no consensus, and protocols regarding specific care vary from physician to physician. Avoid such topics, because you will spend more time discussing whose protocol is best than improving care. A helpful resource for consensus regarding preventive services is the report of the U.S. Preventive Services Task Force, *Guide to Clinical Preventive Services*.

Additional considerations for QI topics include:

- **High cost:** Is there a potential cost benefit? Even if the use of magnetic resonance or computerized tomographic scans is unlikely to be considered common in your practice, a utilization study may point to methods of significant cost savings or improved timing for your patients.
- **High risk:** Even if the condition is uncommon is it considered serious or high risk? The follow-up of abnormal Pap test reports or mammography reports may be required infrequently, but if not done properly it can result in poor patient outcomes and risk of malpractice.
- **Research base:** Is there a clinical research base to help in your development of clinical criteria? Ideally, prospective community-based studies should be available to demonstrate the impact of clinical care on outcomes.

Developing Criteria and Setting Goals

Criteria are statements or guidelines of what your practice considers appropriate patient care. Criteria are not to be used as standards of care from which deviations are inexcusable. Instead, they are yardsticks or gauges against which performance will be measured.

The criteria can be developed by an interested small subgroup of the members of the practice staff. It is useful to limit the scope of the criteria to the most important and the most easily defined or objective aspects of medical care.

> *Example:* Breast cancer screening in your practice could be identified as the topic of interest. The generally accepted criteria include adequate breast self-examinations, clinical breast examinations, and mammograms, all at different time intervals. This could become too involved for any small group. An appropriately focused CQI project could analyze the frequency of mammograms in women aged 50 and above.

Criteria should reflect current knowledge, experience, and guidelines of care for a particular medical problem. Because the problems being reviewed are usually familiar to family physicians and clinical staff, criteria can often be developed from our working knowledge and experience. However, it is valuable to have criteria that are well supported by the literature and that have a solid clinical research base. Criteria can be adapted from the practice guidelines developed and published by professional organizations such as the American College of Obstetrics and Gynecology or the National Cholesterol Education Program. Literature reviews, local practitioners' experiences, and the opinions of local experts or specialists can be used to supplement or amend published guidelines.

The criteria should be put into a format that is conducive to review: simple, clear, objective, and with a yes/no answer. It is important to present the criteria to everyone who provides or participates in care. Consensus before care is measured is a key difference between CQI and QI.

The setting of goals is important in the consensus statement. Goals will vary between institutions and depend on the importance of the process in patient outcomes, the resources of the clinic, and the patients receiving care.

> *Example:* A goal of 80% compliance with mammography in women over age 50 would be a huge improvement in most clinic settings. However, only 100% compliance would be acceptable for "further evaluation of a woman with a suspicious lesions on mammogram" or

"a smoker with a nodule on chest X ray." Goals can also be formulated in terms of improvement—a 10% improvement in compliance in the next 3 months.

Measuring Care

Once the topic, criteria, and goals have been selected the next step is to determine what data are needed and how they should be collected. The steps include selecting a patient sample, developing a review form, performing the review, and presenting the results.

The sample selected will depend on the topic and how you choose to focus it. The sample can be defined by groupings such as:

1. Diagnosis or visit type
   Annual physical exam, urinary tract infection, cough
   New patient, established patient, brief, extended
2. Age
   Child < than 18 years, very elderly > 85 years, or age 40 to 50
3. Gender
4. Combinations of the above
   Female children in for routine exams

The outcome of your study is dependent on appropriate selection of the sample. For example, studying influenza vaccinations in a sample selected by diagnosis may be very different than in a sample selected by age. Those people over 65 seen for chronic pulmonary conditions should have a higher goal for influenza vaccination than merely those seen at age greater than 65.

Once sample selection criteria are agreed upon, then a method of sampling and the number of charts or encounters to be included in the sample can be defined. Samples can be 100% time samples. This means reviewing all patients or encounters in some specified time period that meet the age, diagnosis, or other selection criteria. A systematic sample can be every 3rd or 10th patient seen, or every 20th chart on the record shelf. This type of sample selection is not acceptable for research studies but is perfectly acceptable for internal CQI. Random sampling is of course also acceptable.

Table 21.2 Confidence Intervals for Various Sample Sizes for a Confidence Coefficient of 95%

20 cases	±18%
50 cases	±11%
100 cases	± 7%

Deciding how many charts to review will depend on your resources, the importance of the topic, and the number of potential sample members. The sample size needs to be sufficient to give an accurate assessment of what really happens in the clinic. A few charts may give you an idea of what is happening in your practice but it is useful to be a little more precise. The precision or accuracy of a measurement can be denoted by the confidence interval that surrounds the measurement. The confidence interval (CI) is written as 80% +/− 12%, or 80% and CI 95 (68% to 92%). This means that, considering the number of charts you reviewed, it can be stated with 95% assurance that the actual percentage falls between 68% and 92%. Some rules of thumb can help you decide on the number of cases you must review and what confidence interval you will accept.

In general, the confidence intervals for various sample sizes for a confidence coefficient of 95% are shown in Table 21.2. If your compliance goal for doing mammograms is 90% it would make little sense to allow your variation to be ±18% or even ±11%. Therefore you would have to examine at least 100 charts if you choose goals this high. In very small or young practices you may have to settle for smaller sample sizes and less assurance of your accuracy.

CQI projects should not require new data sources or new methods to collect data. It is important to know what resources you have and to use the CQI work group to decide how best to obtain useful data. Common data sources include patient charts, encounter or billing forms, incident reports, laboratory reports, and radiology reports. Some computerized billing systems can print lists of patients with a specific diagnosis or certain demographic characteristics such as gender and age.

Name	Date	Provider	Mammogram recommended	If not, last mammogram < 1 year (yes/no)
1				
2				
3				
4				
5				
Totals				

Patient name: _____

Date: _____

Provider: _____

	Yes	No
Mammogram recommended	____	____
If no, last mammogram < 1 year	____	____

Figure 21.2. Examples of Data Collection Forms

Data or practice information must be collected on standardized forms. The form should be very simple and very clear. A separate form can be completed for each patient or all information can be placed on a single form. The single form makes summary of the data simpler. Two examples of data forms are shown in Figure 21.2.

The actual data collection can be done by anyone who has the time, access to the data source, and any necessary clinical expertise. It may be best to leave the collection to someone who is not directly providing the type of care to be assessed.

Results

Presenting the results of the data collection is a critical step in CQI. It must be clear what the topic is, what criteria were used, what goals were desired, and the summary of the data collected. Data should never be presented as the final analysis.

Improving Care

The first question must always be: Does care need to be improved? If the data show that your group has matched the goals set for the criteria of care you established then no change is demanded. However, in most projects you will not meet the initial goals. Concern about the care is usually the reason you did the project in the first place. Rather than assuming any care is at fault, it is best to do a diagnostic evaluation. Play with the data. Is there a large variation among providers? Did you fail to account for variations in patient population among providers? Can you identify other factors that might explain the data; for example, mammography is seldom recommended on Mondays when providers are especially busy.

This part of the process is often the most stimulating and most likely to engage the attention of everybody in the practice. The work group is the first place to present the results. Many of these people are closely involved in the topic area and may have insights to provide. Don't make the mistake of discussing the results with only the direct care providers. It is often the receptionists or lab technicians who have the answers to how the system works, what barriers might exist, and why the variations exist. The discussion that ensues will provide insight into the way care is delivered and will present opportunities for improvement. Sometimes a more complete and formal evaluation and assessment of the process of care is needed to shed light on where the system is breaking down.

The final decisions on how to improve care will depend on the hypothesized reasons for the problems. Seldom is a single method of improvement sufficient. The common methods to improve the system are feedback (either group or individual), education, and system changes.

Group feedback is the most effective method for explaining what has been done in the CQI process and what is left to do to meet the defined goals. The feedback should be done in a nonthreatening way and can even be presented in a newsletter or other informational sheet given to all employees. Individual feedback may be interpreted as accusatory and should be done carefully and in a confidential manner. Individuals can then make changes as they desire.

Education is occasionally helpful, especially if the process being assessed involves newly reported recommendations or a change in local or current standards of care. But 85% of quality problems are caused by system failures and system change may be the best approach to problem solving. System change requires the same type of process used to identify criteria. Work groups of interested employees can meet to identify the components of the system and to look for barriers that may exist. Methods to remove barriers or facilitate solutions can come from any and all members of the staff.

Example:
Pediatric Eye Care

Topic Selection

The kindergarten school screening reports sent to the office reported two children with marked visual impairment that had not been previously recognized. One child had severe myopia and the other had amblyopia with severely impaired vision in one eye. Review of their records and discussion with the consulting ophthalmologist revealed that the amblyopia should have been recognized by at least age 3 and if recognized and treated could have prevented vision loss. The severe myopia should have been recognized on the preschool exam; early treatment may have helped the child adjust more quickly to her new surroundings in school.

Criteria and Goal Selection

The practice staff wonder if vision is routinely screened. The medical literature recommends vision screening of all children at ages 3 and 5. You establish visual acuity and amblyopia screening at ages 3 and 5 as your criteria and desire a goal of 95% compliance.

Table 21.3 Data Summary for Pediatric Eye Care Example

Provider	Acuity Screen	Amblyopia Screen	Both Screens
1	12/12 (100%)	12/12 (100%)	12/12 (100%)
2	1/8 (12%)	0/8 (0%)	0/8 (0%)
3	7/14 (50%)	3/14 (21%)	3/14 (21%)
4	1/6 (17%)	0/6 (0%)	0/6 (0%)
Totals	21/40 (52%)	15/40 (38%)	15/40 (38%)

Data Collection and Data Summary

Your data collection form simply records whether vision screening is done at least once before age 6. Your sample is all children age 6 who are registered in your practice and have been seen at least once in the past 3 years. The data summary is presented in Table 21.3.

Results

The results were presented to the work group, who thought that they should be shared with the entire group and that all the providers should receive a confidential report on their patients compared to the group averages and the goals.

Improving Care

Follow-up discussion revealed that not all providers were aware of the need for vision screening, assuming that it was done elsewhere on all children. Most nurses did not know how to do testing on young children. Current scheduling policy did not allow time for this additional testing.

Educational sessions were conducted to explain testing for amblyopia and visual acuity in young children. The sessions were attended by nursing, medical, and receptionist staff members.

The system was changed to allow an extra 5 minutes for well-child exams on 3- and 5-year-olds; nurses automatically completed this testing while rooming the patient.

Providers had the results to interpret and make referrals when appropriate at the time of the exam.

Remeasuring

It is inappropriate to assume that your actions in improving care have been successful. Remeasuring is essential to the CQI process. It is the "continuous" part of the CQI equation. You need to document your improvement and make further modifications if necessary. Remeasuring should occur several times after the initial project to assure that changes are valid and continue to be maintained. Remeasuring is done using the same criteria and methods as the initial assessment. If you achieve your goals and maintain them through at least one or two "remeasures" you may want to close the process and move on to new topics. If you cannot achieve your goals after two or three improvement cycles it is time to reassess your goals and consider an outside opinion.

No one enjoys paperwork, but it is important to document what you do in each step of the CQI process. In addition to having this documentation available to outside groups requesting "quality" data, the careful documentation will be useful in future CQI projects.

As you become more proficient in CQI you may wish to expand your capabilities. Several books and papers are available to teach you techniques such as Pareto or fishbone analysis and are included in the references.

There are two drawbacks of the CQI technique that practitioners should recognize. The first is that this is a process of incremental change, building and changing the current system. If your system requires drastic organizational or structural changes, do not attempt to use the CQI process. The second problem is that the CQI process does not tell you what to do or what goals to attempt. For example, you could use this process to perfect your hospital's open cholecystectomy service, when what you really should be doing is learning laparoscopic techniques. To avoid these problems, it is important to avoid narrowing the focus of the study too early in the process.

References

Berwick, D. M. (1989). Continuous improvement as an ideal in health care. *New England Journal of Medicine, 320,* 53-56.

A short article that compares and contrasts CQI and QI and describes the fundamental requirements for CQI in health care.

Berwick, D. M., & Godfrey, B. A. (1990). *Curing health care: New strategies for quality improvement.* San Francisco: Jossey-Bass.

This book outlines the vision of CQI in medicine based on work with the national demonstration project on quality improvement in health care.

Fisher, M. (Ed.). (1989). *Guide to clinical preventive services.* Baltimore, MD: Williams & Wilkins.

The report of the U.S. Preventive Services Task Force. Should be in every medical library including yours.

Goldfield, N., & Nash, D. B. (Eds.). (1989). *Providing quality care.* Philadelphia: American College of Physicians.

Joint Commission on Accreditation of Healthcare Organizations (JCAHO). (1990). *Quality assurance in ambulatory care* (2nd ed.). Chicago: Author.

Describes the 10-step monitoring and evaluation method of QI.

Joint Commission on Accreditation of Healthcare Organizations (JCAHO). (1992). *The guide to surveying small and rural hospitals.* Oakbrook Terrace, IL: Author.

James, B. C. (1989). *Quality management for health care.* Chicago: Hospital Research and Educational Trust.

A manual for QI in the hospital setting with concepts pertinent to the ambulatory setting.

McCoy, C. E., & Harper, P. G. (Eds.). (1992). *The family practice guide to quality improvement.* Minneapolis: Minnesota Academy of Family Physicians. (Available from the Minnesota Academy of Family Physicians, 2221 University Avenue SE, Suite 426, Minneapolis, MN 55414; phone 1-800-999-8198)

Resources

JCAHO
875 Michigan Avenue
Chicago, IL 60611

Hospital Research and Education Trust
American Hospital Association
840 North Lake Shore Drive
Chicago, IL 60611

22
■ ■ ■

Living Through Malpractice Litigation

J. RANDALL RAUH

ANGELINE BUSHY

Introduction

Information about the human dimension of medical litigation is sparse, particularly as it relates to physicians who practice in rural environments. Stemming from demographic, cultural, and socioeconomic factors, physician-community dynamics in rural areas differ from those in more populated settings (Weinert & Long, 1991). This chapter will address the impact of litigation on rural physicians. The information presented here is based on the literature, observing and talking with rural physicians and other health care providers who have been involved with the legal system, interviews with lawyers, and our personal experiences of living and working in rural environments, and our testimony as expert witnesses for cases involving rural health care providers.

Rationale

The purpose of this discussion is threefold: (a) to create awareness among physicians of the human response to the personal crisis of litigation with its associated losses and grieving; (b) to disseminate information and provide guidance and emotional support to physicians should they become involved with the legal system; and (c) to provide a reference source that can be used to validate feelings and responses of physicians who are or have been involved in

AUTHOR'S NOTE: Adapted from Bushy, A., & Rauh, J. (1993). The human response to professional litigation in rural practice: Application of Caplan's theory of crisis. *Family and Community Health, 16*(1), 55-66.

litigation, particularly those in more isolated, rural practice settings (Caplan, 1981; Charles, Wilbert, & Kennedy, 1984; Kuhlman, 1990). A significant number of physicians will be involved in litigation at some time during their professional careers. A practitioner can be sued no matter how skilled he or she may be, and many have found themselves unexpectedly in court. The literature indicates that regardless of the practice setting (rural vs. urban), physicians are at risk of medical litigation. In urban areas, specialty is a major determinant of physician risk. Yet, rural physicians often are geographically and professionally isolated. Insufficient numbers of professionals practice in most rural areas. This deficit often mandates that rural providers function with greater autonomy and in expanded roles. With more responsibilities, there are increased risks for maloccurrence and hence a greater potential for litigation (McQuade, 1991; Rauh, 1991; Ward, 1991).

Involvement with the legal system may assume broader dimensions in rural practice. For instance, a patient also may be one's neighbor, relative, friend, or a member of the same church organizations. These close personal relationships can result in some unusual circumstances for rural physicians involved in litigation, their families, peers, and associates, and the community as a whole.

It is not unusual for a doctor who is sued to describe this event as a personal and professional crisis (Holmes & Rahe, 1967). Dealing with a crisis is easier if it can be put in a framework and responses and actions are anticipated. In this chapter, medical litigation will be discussed within the framework of Caplan's Crisis Theory (Caplan, 1961, 1964, 1981).

Caplan's Theory of Crisis

A crisis is defined by Caplan (1964) as a short period of disequilibrium in an individual who confronts a hazardous circumstance, serious life disruption, or an important problem. The person can neither escape nor solve the event with customary problem-solving skills. Crisis always involves some kind of change, resulting in a rise in inner tension. The resultant stress is manifested by symptoms of anxiety, confusion, inability to function, and extended periods of emotional upset (Holmes & Rahe, 1967).

There are always losses in a crisis. For physicians who are sued, losses may include financial loss, personal integrity, professional status, career ideals, personal goals, and changes in relationships. Loss does not occur in isolation. Rather, it has a ripple effect that disrupts many other aspects of the physician's life. Most crisis and grief reactions do not require outside intervention. Generally, informal support systems such as family, friends, clergy, and peers are quite effective in helping a person through the critical events.

Caplan's model can be a useful framework to assist physicians in handling the crises of litigation. He identifies four phases in a crisis: *impact, disorganization, recovery,* and *reorganization.* Each of these has characteristic feelings and responses. Even though the model is depicted as linear and systematic, the actual process may not always proceed in this manner. Depending upon personal coping style and perceived resources, most individuals work through a crisis in an irregular process. They may progress, regress, then advance toward reorganization, or remain fixed in a particular phase. For some the resolution of a crisis may extend over years, even an entire lifetime. Keeping in mind the circular nature of crisis resolution, the subsequent discussion highlights characteristic behaviors for each phase in a crisis (Table 22.1).

Phase I: Impact

In Phase I the person becomes aware of the crisis. Characteristic human responses to the disruption are shock, numbness, disbelief, and denial. A person may express feelings of unreality, confusion, turmoil, and uncertainty. Customary coping strategies often do not work to resolve the issue, causing the person to feel even more upset. The problem persists, forcing a person to become aware of the personal and professional magnitude of the crisis.

Phase II: Disorganization

The problem persists and disorganization becomes evident, characterized by feelings of stress, hopelessness, increased tension, depression, conflict, and anxiety. Somatic complaints are common, especially symptoms of insomnia, gastrointestinal disturbances, upper respiratory infections, fatigue, headaches, and backaches.

Table 22.1 Characteristic Human Responses During a Crisis

Phase I Impact ⟷	Phase II Disorganization ⟷	Phase III Recovery ⟷	Phase IV Reorganization
Numbness	Increased tension	Active coping	Changing
Disbelief	Depression	Constructive behaviors	Adapting
Denial	Conflict	Destructive behaviors	Integrating
Unreality	Hopelessness	Scapegoating	
Shock	Anxiety	Minimizing	
Trauma	Evolving awareness	Intellectualizing	
	Isolation	Being strong	
	Shame	Blaming	
	Doubt	Repeating	
	Guilt	Negative expectations	
	Anger	Self-medicating	
	Powerlessness	Depersonalization	
	Suicidal ideation	Finding meaning	
	Somatic complaints	Somatic complaints	

SOURCE: Adapted from: Caplan, 1964; Kübler-Ross, 1969; Martin, Wilson, Fielbelman, Gurley, & Miller, 1991.

The symptoms may be self-treated with over-the-counter and self-prescribed prescription medications, even samples provided to the doctor by drug companies.

To address the overwhelming situation, the affected person augments usual problem-solving methods with novel coping approaches. Coping behaviors can be construed to be either constructive (healthy) or detrimental (unhealthy) depending upon the outcome(s) for the physician. To assess the "healthiness" of a coping behavior, the action should be considered in relation to the impact on the person who uses it, the frequency with which the behavior is used, and the effect on the person's family, peers, and community (Kübler-Ross, 1969; Lindemann, 1965; Satir, 1967).

For instance, behaviors that may be viewed as more constructive include seeking support from family or friends, getting more involved in work, participating in religious or spiritual practices, and increasing physical activity. Behaviors that may be detrimental include indiscriminate use of alcohol, mood alternating drugs, sleeping pills, and over-the-counter or sample-prescription medications to treat somatic complaints; social and professional isolation; physical and verbal aggression; overeating; and neglecting or exploiting a particular family member, peer, or friend. Many physicians engage in less obvious, more subtle mechanisms such as minimizing, intellectualizing, repeating, and "acting strong" to cope with the overwhelming anxiety and the painful reality of litigation.

Minimizing is characterized by a reduction of, or attempt to ignore, the significance of the event. This behavior is more evident in the early stages of the crisis, evidenced by cheerful nonchalance or an inability to remember pertinent information. *Intellectualizing* is an overly rational attitude about the event, evidenced by discussing technical aspects of the case and avoiding the emotional component. *Repetition* in speech can be a form of avoidance, allowing one to focus on the more tolerable and to avoid the more painful aspects of the event. Or it can be a way to validate and confront reality while gradually assimilating the stressful facts of an event.

When *acting strong*, the affected person presents a demeanor of competency, control, and ability to deal with the crisis event. Peers and patients may view this survival response as arrogance and respond in an antagonistic manner. However, this coping behavior also can provide secondary gains. As a family and community member, it is not unusual for the strong one to be the leader and spokesperson during a crisis. Likewise, the strong role can be a source of personal satisfaction while serving as a model for family pride and leadership and inspire others to assume new responsibilities with greater enthusiasm.

Coping behaviors such as minimizing, intellectualizing, repetition, and acting strong can reduce tension and allow for more effective crisis resolution on a temporary basis. The feelings of helplessness, guilt, and the somatic symptoms are cyclic and will continue to reemerge for some time. The turning point of a crisis takes place when the internal tension mobilizes previously hidden strengths, making it possible to begin recovery.

Phase III: Recovery

With recovery, the disorganization is overcome by the struggle to identify a reason or meaning for the disruption. Generally, feelings of depression persist until the person has achieved satisfactory insight about the events. Long-term struggles with psychologic symptoms or incapacitation indicate that a negative meaning has been attributed to the experience, such as punishment for one's misdeeds, bad luck, or blaming another person. Examples of positive interpretations for a crisis include acknowledging personal responsibility for life events and recognizing the importance of those experiences in the maturation process.

Phase IV: Reorganization

Once a positive or negative meaning has been given to the event, reorganization begins. The person comes to terms with the problem and starts to feel in control of life. The individual integrates the disruption and losses into his or her life views and is impatient for life to return to normal, even though he or she is unsure what constitutes the postcrisis normal state. Ultimately, a physician who has been sued should perceive the event to be one of many types of events that must be mastered and incorporated into a practice.

Caplan's Theory Applied to the Family and Community

A crisis-producing situation affects not only the person who is directly involved, but also family, friends, and peers (Caplan, 1961, 1964; Satir, 1967). The community must also come to terms with the fact that a local physician is being sued. Caplan's model is also appropriate for groups because they experience a crisis in much the same manner as an individual. Upon impact, a family and community feel shock and numbness to the disruption, refusing to believe that a problem exists or intellectualizing acceptance without any emotional involvement. As the facts are assimilated, there is a downward slump in the group's organizational function. A group exhibits a wide range of emotional responses that are reflected in its approach to the involved physician.

A group may avoid or emotionally isolate the person who is directly affected. Or, there may be role shifting by certain individuals in order to adapt to the changes and to maintain some degree of stability within the group. Unusual coping behaviors may increase group tension. As recovery takes place, lasting changes occur within the group as it reorganizes and gives meaning to the disrupting events. Unfortunately, the community may become involved in the problem long after the physician and his or her family and peers have begun the resolution process. This may trigger a new crisis for those affected.

Human Responses to Medical Litigation

Although the patterns of response to medical litigation mesh with Caplan's four-phase crisis theory, the response to the event varies from person to person. Responses depend on the person's coping skills and the quantity and quality of his or her social support (Charles, 1988; Charles et al., 1984; Charles, Wilbert, & Franke, 1985; Martin, Wilson, Fiebelman, Gurley, & Miller, 1991). The effect on the community may depend on the longevity of the physician in the community, the depth to which the physician has integrated into the community structure, and the perceived need of this community for the physician's services. The remaining discussion focuses on the responses of rural physicians to illustrate better the human side of medical litigation.

The Impact of Receiving the Subpoena

The telephone rings. "It's your wife," says the office nurse. I answer it. My wife tells me, "The county sheriff has been at our house three times today—in full uniform—looking for you. He informed me he has a subpoena for a malpractice suit that was filed by a former patient of yours." Out of courtesy to my patients, I suppose, the sheriff did not come to my office to serve the legal documents. Since my work hours at the clinic were extremely long, he made several home visits before waiting outside of my office for me one evening to give me the subpoena. I also received a letter by certified mail. It said: Please be advised that a proposed complaint of malpractice has been filed with the U.S. Federal Court of . . . naming me as a defendant. The shock sets in; my body goes numb—except for the pounding of my heart. Getting the subpoena was bad enough; but, the daily sight of the sheriff in full uniform coming up to my home to question the children as to my whereabouts took its toll on them. I experienced this unpleasant shock in spring of 1979 and the trial was held in early 1981. Two years is a rather short time compared to other medical malpractice cases, which often end up in the court system for a decade or longer. During that time, my acute anxiety changed to chronic concern. These feelings intensified whenever I received correspondence from my lawyers, the insurance company, read about similar malpractice cases and attended a legal seminar. To this day, my family and I continue to feel the effects of this event.

From this physician, one can appreciate the impact of receiving a notice of a malpractice suit. But that is only the beginning of a long, drawn out process.

The Legal Process Exacerbates Disorganization

The physical and emotional effects of the long-term stress is evident in the following remarks:

> Following the arrival of the subpoena, my workload increased. This probably was a kind of self-induced therapy; perhaps, a form of denial to not work through the grieving process. Certainly, my family and office staff experienced the immediate effects of my anger and denial. As the weeks passed, I experienced significant weight loss, menstrual changes, anorexia, irritability, and insomnia. For a time, I became seriously depressed and sought professional help. The depression has abated but, on occasion, cynicism and apathy are still evident. As a specialist it was, and sometimes still is, difficult for me to accept referrals from other practitioners in our multi-county catchment area.

Symptoms of depression can have a cyclic effect on one's relationships, work, and leisure activities. Depression disrupts the ability to concentrate, impairing a physician's clinical and decision-making skills, even increasing the physician's risk for future maloccurrence. The next quotation exemplifies the spiraling effects of depression on family and peers:

> After I received the [legal] papers, things went down hill for me, personally as well as in my practice. My wife was devastated by the legal proceedings and became extremely depressed. We did not directly involve our children in any of the discussions regarding the case. Yet, they never resolved the question as to whether or not their father did something really bad enough to be pursued by the legal authorities. Ultimately, after 23 years of marriage, my wife filed for a divorce, resulting in yet another crisis.

Dissolution of marriage may not occur in every situation, but the prevailing uncertainty and the length of time to finalize a legal case

impose extreme stress on marital and family relationships. Ultimately the outcome of a relationship depends on a couple's short-
and long-term coping skills, as litigation is an emotionally intensive
and exhausting process. In particular, the information-seeking activity on the part of lawyers known as *discovery* may take a heavy
toll on the physician. In the next passage, by Mullen (1991), one can
observe how the process of discovery exacerbates disorganization,
especially for physicians who live and work in a small, close-knit
town:

> This bruising, bare knuckle prelude to a trial, known to lawyers by
> the mild-mannered term "discovery," describes the initial stages of a
> lawsuit in which each side gathers evidence, postures, bluffs, plots
> strategy and measures the other side's chances for victory. Discovery
> means exactly what it implies; both sides seek to uncover evidence to
> bolster their case or damage the opposition's to use in the subtle art of
> negotiations . . . finding useful dirt. Critics say the discovery task has
> turned the court's task from weighing justice to brokering settle-
> ments, mainly for insurance companies.

Coping With the Litigation Process

Some cases are settled out of court whereas others require a trial;
but whatever the outcome, the ongoing uncertainty is painful for all
involved, as exemplified by this physician's remarks:

> My trial was rescheduled four or five times. My wife accompanied me
> to the courthouse each time. The uncertainty was emotionally devas-
> tating for both of us. In the end the case was tried as a product liability
> as opposed to medical practice. The jury gave the plaintiff $60,000
> divided among the three defendants; myself, the drug distributor, and
> the product manufacturer. Considering that they originally asked for
> $1.2 million, this outcome might be viewed as a victory of sorts.
> Compared to the pain endured by my family and me during this
> process, I find little consolation in the low judgment award.

Recovery

As with other situational crises, recovery eventually occurs, but
seldom before litigation is completed. Because a case can be tied
up in the courts for years; this can hinder resolution by the person, family, and community. After a final legal decision has been

reached, reorganization can begin. This phase of crisis resolution frequently requires decision making. Are you willing to continue practicing in your discipline? Will you modify previous practice patterns, and if so, how? Most physicians do continue practicing and most become more realistic about the potential for litigation. Physicians are usually most comfortable when helping others. Recovery may be facilitated by helping other physicians and families deal with malpractice and the personal, professional, and family upheaval that even the threat of a lawsuit may cause:

> I thought I had dealt with the lawsuit and my feelings. When the medical association asked me to be part of a program about malpractice I agreed willingly. We were about 10 minutes into the 2-hour session when the panic hit. Most of my colleagues were unaware of the malpractice suit settled out of court 5 years earlier. Everyone else on the panel had been to trial and had been vindicated, while I agreed to settle out of court. The total award from five physicians and the hospital was $50,000 to be paid over 5 years, but unlike my peers I had not been vindicated. My recovery process began that day. My colleagues accepted me and continue to support me.

Community Impact and Disorganization

Because there are fewer people in small rural communities, many of whom are personally acquainted, an untoward event that affects a local person soon becomes common knowledge (Brodsky, 1991; Rauh, 1991; Weinert & Long, 1991). Malpractice claims usually become the center of attention for residents living in a small town, especially when a public announcement is made by the local media. Local news reports usually explain a case in some detail, including the names of prosecutors, defendants, and sometimes lawyers. The ripple effects of public reports combined with informal communication patterns are described by the next report:

> Historically, malpractice claims were rarely reported by the local media. However, the case for which I was subpoenaed was a break from tradition. Details of my malpractice charge were reported on the front page of our small town newspaper and then quoted during a newscast by our local radio station. I queried the newspaper editor regarding their change in policy regarding locally filed claims. He explained that I was highly active in the community; therefore, seen as a public

figure. From his view, legal actions involving public figures, in this case me, were newsworthy and deserved being reported . . . more so than if one has less community visibility. Following the public announcements, the townsfolk changed. Friends as well as acquaintances subtly raised questions. Perhaps I had actually done something wrong. Why else would a lawsuit have been filed? Constantly, I encounter innuendos and outright accusations of being a provider of poor care. I have become quite sensitive to those remarks. Unfortunately, the public repercussions are also directed toward my family, which increases the stress at home. In a small town it is extremely difficult for a physician to distance oneself from the friends and family of persons who filed the claim. For me, as the only surgeon in a three-county area, there are numerous opportunities to treat family members of the plaintiff and his attorney.

Impact of Litigation on Medical Practice

Involvement with the legal system necessitates changes in a physician's practice (Charles et al., 1984; Charles et al., 1985; Kuhlman, 1990; Martin et al., 1991). Another rural doctor comments on the unanticipated logistic and financial problems that are associated with litigation:

> Being the only doctor in a 90-mile radius created serious logistic and financial problems for me each time I left town to provide depositions and to attend the trial. In addition to the inconvenience and cost of not working and traveling, I had to arrange for locum tenens (temporary, short-term replacement) to cover my practice while I was gone. Outside of the legal expenses paid by the insurance company, my out-of-pocket costs for the case approached $55,000.

Peer Responses to Litigation:
Physicians and Nurses

Litigation influences peer relationships, especially in an underserved community. Within a few days after a local doctor receives a subpoena, practice patterns become more cautious, hesitant, and defensive. Physicians who have been sued may contact the recently subpoenaed peer and talk openly about their experiences. Their conversations often include gallows humor and rarely do they openly express feelings about the day-to-day, emotional impact of litiga-

314 EXPLORING RURAL MEDICINE

tion. Physicians who have never been sued may distance themselves from a peer who is currently dealing with this crisis. One
physician described her peers' behavior in this way: "They avoid
me . . . I feel if they talk to me, they might catch something serious."
Litigation affects relationships with other types of health providers. One physician noted that his relationship with the nurses who
worked in the local hospital changed dramatically following litigation. Some of the new nursing behaviors could be classified as
excellent risk-management strategies; but others inhibited interdisciplinary rapport, and therefore impaired care. Nurses who had
previously been summoned as court witnesses demonstrated varying degrees of concern regarding patients' motives. Overall, locally
filed cases can create barriers to effective interdisciplinary practice
in rural environments.

Helping Families Cope

From the first hint of a malpractice suit, the physician's family is
affected. Family members and friends are often frightened and frus-
trated, and feel inadequate during the long process of medical litigation (Caplan, 1981; Charles, 1988; Kübler-Ross, 1969; Kuhlman,
1990; Lindemann, 1965). Family and friends need permission to
help and guidance from the physician or a supportive colleague.

- Let them know it is all right to talk about the event.
- If someone offers to help, suggest specific tasks for which the physician and spouse have no energy (e.g., errands, answering the phone,
  social responsibilities).
- Children need special attention. Ask their friends or special adults in
  their lives to help support them.
- Let them know that someone must continue to listen, even though
  the story or feelings may be repetitious.
- Tell them the need for emotional support may increase after several
  months when the reality sets in, and feelings of isolation, guilt, and
  lack of confidence are evident.
- Reassure the participants that they should not be embarrassed to cry,
  get angry, or express negative emotions with family and friends.
- Encourage them to respect their feelings and needs; bring them out
  into the open by expressing them to a person who is trustworthy,
  understanding, and accepting.

Physicians are vulnerable during the extended legal process. They will need the following:

- Respect and dignity
- Information
- Help in consideration of options and choices
- Safety, but not necessarily protection
- Support in communicating losses (real and perceived)
- People physically present to offer support and encouragement
- An understanding of the normalcy of the grief response
- Distraction and an occasional chance to get away
- Focus on the experience of litigation and its meaning in life
- Opportunity to experience life events unrelated to the legal issue
- Association with friends or persons who know them, accept whatever they are feeling, and affirm their belief in themselves and their abilities
- Contact with other people who have had a similar experience and are willing to share insights and give hope (a support group with other physicians who have been sued)
- Recollection of personal strengths evidenced in previous times of difficulty or stress
- Encouragement, love, and affection

Summary

There is no sure protection against medical litigation. In the event that this situation does occur, Caplan's theory of crisis can serve as a useful framework to help a physician and his or her family cope with the events surrounding the case.

References

Brodsky, S. (1991). Jury selection in malpractice suits: An investigation into community attitudes toward malpractice and physicians. *International Journal of Law & Psychiatry, 14*(3), 215-219.

Caplan, G. (1961). *An approach to community mental health.* New York: Grune & Stratton.

Caplan, G. (1964). *Principles of preventive psychiatry.* New York: Basic Books.

Caplan, G. (1981). Mastery of stress: Psychosocial aspects. *American Journal of Psychiatry, 138,* 413-427.

Charles, S., Wilbert, J., & Kennedy, E. (1984). Physicians' self reports of reactions to malpractice litigation. *American Journal of Psychiatry, 141,* 563-565.

Charles, S., Wilbert, J., & Franke, K. (1985). Sued and non-sued physicians' reported reactions to malpractice litigation. *American Journal of Psychiatry, 142,* 437-442.

Charles, S. (1988). Psychological reactions to medical malpractice suits and the development of support groups as a response. *Instructor Course Lecture, 37,* 289-292.

Holmes, T., & Rahe, R. (1967). The social readjustment rating scale. *Journal of Psychometric Research, 11,* 213-218.

Kübler-Ross, E. (1969). *On death and dying.* New York: Macmillan.

Kuhlman, C. (1990). Surviving a malpractice suit: Personal experience and general information. *Journal of Nursing Midwifery, 35*(3), 166-171.

Lindemann, E. (1965). Symptomatology and management of acute grief. In H. Parad (Ed.), *Crisis intervention: Selected readings* (pp. 101, 121-143). New York: Family Association of America.

Martin, C., Wilson, J., Fiebelman, N., Gurley, D., & Miller, T. (1991). Physicians' psychological reactions to malpractice litigation. *Southern Medical Journal, 84* (11), 1300-1304.

McQuade, J. (1991). The medical malpractice crisis—Reflections on the alleged causes and proposed cures. *Journal of Rural Sociology & Medicine, 84*(7), 408-411.

Mullen, W. (1991, August 4-7). Lawsuit craze turns liability into high-stake lottery [4-part series]. *The Salt Lake Tribune,* pp. 1-2.

Rauh, J. (1991). Medical malpractice: A rural obstetrician's perspective. In A. Bushy (Ed.), *Rural nursing-Vol. I* (pp. 150-165). Newbury Park, CA: Sage.

Satir, V. (1967). *Conjoint family therapy.* Palo Alto, CA: Science Association of America.

Ward, C. (1991). Analysis of 500 obstetric and gynecologic malpractice claim cases and prevention. *American Journal of Obstetrics Gynecology, 165*(2), 304-306.

Weinert, C., & Long, K. (1991). The theory and research base for rural nursing practice. In A. Bushy (Ed.), *Rural nursing-Vol. I* (pp. 21-38). Newbury Park, CA: Sage.

Index

About the Authors

Angeline Bushy, RN, PhD, received a BSN in nursing at the University of Mary in Bismarck, North Dakota; an MN in Community Health Nursing from Montana State University; an MEd in Adult Education from Northern Montana College; and a PhD in nursing administration and women's health from the University of Texas in Austin. She has published widely and presented nationally and internationally on a variety of topics related to rural nursing. She is the editor of the two-volume text *Rural Nursing* (Sage, 1991). Currently she is Associate Professor of Nursing at the University of Utah College of Nursing in Salt Lake City. Her research interests include body image and women's health and vulnerable rural populations. She has worked in hospitals and community health settings as well as in rural educational institutions.

Daniel D. Broughton, MD, is Associate Professor of Pediatrics and Head of the Community Pediatric Section at Mayo Medical School and Mayo Clinic, Rochester, Minnesota. He attended Georgetown University School of Medicine in Washington, DC, and completed pediatric training at Letterman Army Medical Center in San Francisco. He also is the current Chairman of the Board of Directors of the National Center for Missing and Exploited Children.

Patricia M. Cole, MD, received her medical degree from the University of Minnesota in 1974. She completed a residency in Family Medicine in the Department of Family Practice and Community

Health of the University of Minnesota at Fairview-St. Mary's Hospital in 1977, and a Faculty Development Fellowship at the University of North Carolina in 1990. She is certified by the American Board of Family Practice. She is chairperson for the annual meeting of the Society of Teachers of Family Medicine, and is on the board of directors of that organization. Her special interests are primary care education, especially for residents in educational difficulty; the doctor-patient relationship; organizational diagnosis; and cultural analysis of medical practices. She is currently the director of the family medicine residency at Hennepin County Medical Center in Minneapolis.

Kathy Dubbels, RN, PHN, is a public health nurse for Olmsted County Public Health Services in Minnesota. She has worked as a maternal child health nurse for the past 10 years, spending increasing amounts of time working with Cambodian clients. To establish a basis for understanding the behavior and beliefs of many of her Southeast Asian clients, she has studied the Cambodian culture and worked with local interpreters to develop her expertise.

Charles S. Field, MD, has been actively involved in the clinical practice of obstetrics and gynecology over the past 15 years with a specific interest in obstetrical referral patterns from rural areas. After attending medical school at the University of Minnesota, he completed a residency in obstetrics and gynecology at the Mayo Clinic, Rochester, Minnesota. He subsequently joined the staff of the Mayo Clinic in 1977, serving as Section Head of Obstetrics from 1985 to 1991, and is presently Assistant Professor in Obstetrics and Gynecology in Mayo Medical School. He has been involved in a number of medical organizations including the American College of Obstetrics and Gynecology, the Minnesota State Obstetrical and Gynecological Society, and is currently chairperson of the Minnesota Care Practice Parameter Advisory Committee.

Paul S. Frame, MD, is a family physician in private practice in Dansville, New York, and Cohocton, New York. He is also Clinical Associate Professor in the Department of Family Medicine and the Department of Community and Preventive Medicine at the University of Rochester (New York) School of Medicine and Dentistry, and a member of the U.S. Preventive Services Task Force, a panel commissioned by the Department of Health and Human Services to update preventive recommendations for the practicing physician. He graduated from the University of Pennsylvania School of Medicine and completed a family practice residency at the Hunterton Medical Center, Flemington, New Jersey.

Patricia A. Gibson, PhD, has served as Vice President for Information Services at the American Academy of Family Physicians Foundation, Kansas City, Missouri, since 1983. Previously she worked as a medical librarian in two academic institutions: the University of Oklahoma Health Sciences Center and Wichita State University; and as a hospital librarian at Regional Memorial Hospital in Brunswick, Maine. She received her MLS degree in 1966 and her PhD in 1977, both from the University of Oklahoma. She is a Distinguished Member of the Academy of Health Information Professionals, Medical Library Association. Her special interest in patient education developed from a W. K. Kellogg Foundation grant in health promotion, for which she served as project director from 1986 to 1988.

Peter G. Harper, MD, MPH, is a practicing family physician with the Department of Family Medicine at St. Paul-Ramsey Medical Center in St. Paul, Minnesota, and a member of the Minnesota Academy of Family Physicians Quality Improvement Task Force. He instructs family practice residents in the principles of quality improvement, and manages the QI program for the Family Practice Residency program. He is chairperson of the Ambulatory QI Committee at the Medical Center, and he has participated on several QI teams to enhance patient care while reducing the work load for health care providers. Other active interests include community-oriented primary care and childhood immunizations.

Carole E. Hill, PhD, is from Emory University in Atlanta, Georgia. Her background in anthropology and her many articles and books on the Southern African American culture give her special insight into the importance of cultural awareness in providing health care to this population. In addition to her extensive written works she lectures in medical schools and at medical meetings on how to provide care that will be welcomed and accepted by southern black consumers.

Nancy N. Hoogenhous, MPH, RN, is nurse manager with Children's Respiratory and Critical Care Specialists. She received her Master's in Public Health from the University of Minnesota. She has a special interest in chronic ventilator patients and their families, and her thesis looked at family stress and coping in the home ventilator dependent patient.

Claudia J. Kapp, BA, RNC, is a patient education specialist at the Sioux Falls Family Practice Residency in Sioux Falls, South Dakota. She was the recipient of the 1988 *Patient Care* Award for Excellence in Patient Education. She is certified in Community Health Nursing by the American Nurses Association. She has provided nursing care in a variety of areas including home care, hospital, office and public health. She claims community health nursing as her primary interest. She has developed a curriculum for family practice residents who plan to practice in rural areas; has presented workshops, lectures, and seminars; and has published on the subject of patient education. In addition, she has spoken on patient and community education in the rural setting and has developed an annotated patient education resource file for rural physicians.

David M. Larson, MD, is certified by the American Board of Family Practice, and is in private practice in Northfield, Minnesota. He is medical director of the Northfield Hospital Emergency Department and the Northfield Ambulance Advanced Life Support Services. He serves on the Board of Directors of the Minnesota Association of Emergency Medical Service Physicians, and is a past president of that organization. He is also a member of the Board of Directors of the Minnesota Chapter of the American College of Emergency Physicians, a member of the Minnesota Emergency Medical Services Advisory Council, and Assistant Clinical Professor in the Department of Family Practice and Community Health of the University of Minnesota Medical School.

Charles E. McCoy, MD, is a family physician at Park Nicollet Medical Center in Minneapolis, Minnesota. He is a member of the Minnesota Academy of Family Physicians Task Force on Quality Improvement, and is the coeditor of The Family Practice Guide to Quality Improvement, published by the Academy. He has been medical director of quality assurance for the Park Nicollet Medical Foundation and a surveyor for the Accreditation Association for Ambulatory Health Care. In addition to clinical practice, he is currently medical director for health services research at the Park Nicollet Medical Foundation.

Carolyn McKay, MD, obtained a medical degree from the University of Minnesota and received additional training at the Cleveland Metropolitan General Hospital, the University of Colorado Medical Center, and Johns Hopkins University. She is associated with the University of Minnesota Department of Pediatrics and the School of Public Health. Her practice has included school-based clinics, children with disabilities, children from high-risk pregnancies, underserved rural areas and the non-English speaking population. She has served as administrator of local and state health programs, and is currently the Commissioner of Health for the city of Minneapolis, Minnesota.

John J. McNamara, MD, is a pulmonologist with Children's Respiratory and Critical Care Specialists. He also is Medical Director of Home Care at Minneapolis Children's Medical Center. He received his medical degree at the University of Florida College of Medicine and completed his pediatric residency at the University of Rochester Strong Memorial Hospital in Rochester, New York. He also completed a fellowship in pediatric pulmonology at Boston Children's Hospital and at the Harvard School of Public Health. He was an assistant in medicine at Boston Children's Hospital and an instructor at Harvard Medical School. He is board certified in pediatrics and pediatric pulmonology and has special interests in cystic fibrosis, bronchopulmonary dysplasia, infant pulmonary function, recurrent pneumonias, and congenital malformation of the lung.

Cheri L. Olson, MD, is Associate Director at the St. Francis-Mayo Family Practice Residency in La Crosse, Wisconsin. An Instructor in the Mayo Graduate School of Medicine, she has a particular interest in women's health issues. She lectures widely on contraceptives, menopause, obstetrics, colposcopy, and other gynecological areas for both medical and community groups. She completed a residency and a research fellowship in family medicine at the Mayo

Clinic. She is currently involved in research in areas of women's health.

Lawrence P. Peterson, MD, received his medical degree from the University of Minnesota School of Medicine, and completed a residency in adult psychiatry at the Mayo Graduate School of Medicine. He is certified in adult psychiatry by the American Board of Psychiatry and Neurology. He was a staff psychiatrist at the Rochester State Hospital in Rochester, Minnesota, in 1975-1976, and then practiced at the Minneapolis Clinic of Psychiatry and Neurology until 1978. He was a clinical instructor in psychiatry at the University of Minnesota Medical School from 1978 to 1980, and then joined the Department of Behavioral Medicine of the Gundersen Clinic in LaCrosse, Wisconsin, where he remained until 1990. He is now practicing psychiatry at the Olmsted Medical Group in Rochester, Minnesota, where he is chairperson of the Department of Psychiatry and Psychology. His special interests are neuropsychiatry, attention deficit disorder, religion and psychiatry, medical liaison, and psychopharmacology.

J. Randall Rauh, MD, is a native of rural Oklahoma who received his medical degree from the University of Oklahoma. He completed a residency in obstetrics and gynecology at the University of Oklahoma Tulsa Medical College. He practiced at Okmulgee, Oklahoma, for 5 years before moving to Miles City, Montana, where he has been in practice for 12 years. He is certified by the American Board of Obstetrics and Gynecology and is a Fellow of the American College of Surgeons. He is a Clinical Instructor in obstetrics and gynecology at the University of Oklahoma Tulsa Medical College and a Clinical Instructor in the Department of Community Medicine and Rural Health University of the North Dakota College of Medicine.

Richard D. Simon, Jr., MD, received his medical degree from the University of Chicago Pritzer School of Medicine in 1976. He completed an internal medicine residency at the University of Chicago in 1979 and served as Chief Resident and Instructor in Medicine in 1980. Since 1981 he has practiced general internal medicine in Walla Walla with a special emphasis on HIV infection and AIDS. In 1990 he earned a certificate in biomedical ethics from the University of

Washington. Since 1985 he has organized symposia and given numerous lectures on HIV infection and AIDS directed toward rural primary care providers and persons living in rural areas. He is past President of the Walla Walla Valley Medical Society, past Chairman of Medicine of the Walla Walla Clinic, past Chairman of Medicine of St. Mary's Medical Center in Walla Walla, and is currently Chairman of the CME Committee of St. Mary's Medical Center.

Pelage "Mike" Snesrud, RN, BSN, is a commander in the U.S. Public Health Service and Director of Public Health Nursing at Fond du Lac Reservation. He has 16 years of experience in public health nursing and 13 years in the Indian Health Service. He is a member of the Shakopee Mdewakanton Sioux Community and is heavily involved in working with local, state, and national committees for the achievement of higher levels of health and wellness in the Indian community. He is currently the President of the Indian Health Service National Council of Nurse Administrators and the President of the Alaska Native American Indian Nurses Association.

Wayne H. Thalhuber, MD, is the Medical Director for the Hospice of HealthEast and the Medical Director for Our Lady of Good Counsel Cancer Home in St. Paul, Minnesota. He is certified by the American Board of Internal Medicine and is board eligible in oncology. Because of his interest in palliative care, he has addressed the emerging concept of futile care in medical treatment and has applied this concept to the field of oncology.

Theodore R. Thompson, MD, is Professor of Pediatrics in the Department of Pediatrics at the University of Minnesota. He is currently Director of the Medical Outreach Program for the University of Minnesota Hospital and Clinic, and Associate Chief of Pediatric Services. He was Director of the Division of Neonatology in the Department of Pediatrics at the University of Minnesota from 1977 to 1991. He continues to be actively involved in neonatal medicine, and is treasurer of the Great Plains Organization for Perinatal Health Care. He is also a member of the Board of Directors of Critical Care Services-Life Link III, which provides emergency transport of critically ill patients.

Norma Wylie, MSN, received a master's degree in nursing at the University of California, San Francisco, in 1963. She started the first hospice in eastern Canada in 1976 at Victoria General Hospital, the teaching hospital for Dalhousie University. She joined the faculty of the Departments of Medical Humanities and Surgery at Southern Illinois University in 1978. She developed and taught an elective course on death and dying at the Southern Illinois University School of Medicine from 1979 to 1985. She served on the planning committee for St. John's Hospice in Springfield, Illinois, from 1979 to 1982. In 1980 she published *The Role of the Nurse in Medical Education.*

Barbara P. Yawn, MD, MS, became the Coordinator of Clinical Research at the Olmsted Medical Group in Rochester, Minnesota in 1992. Before assuming that position she was a full-time family physician for 12 years in a rural practice in Worthington, Minnesota. In addition to her interests in rural clinical research and perinatal practice, she has been a preceptor for family practice residents in South Dakota, Wisconsin, and Minnesota. She has spoken nationally and internationally and has published papers about teen sexuality, patient education, preterm labor, and other topics of interest to rural physicians. In 1988 she received the *Patient Care* Award for Excellence in Patient Education at the Tenth Annual Conference on Patient Education in the Primary Care Setting at Kansas City, Missouri. She earned the Outstanding Scientific Paper Award of the American Academy of Family Physicians at the Annual Assemblies in both 1988 and 1989.

Roy A. Yawn, MD, obtained his medical degree at the University of Missouri in Columbia, and completed a residency in internal medicine at the University of Minnesota. He is board certified by the American Board of Internal Medicine in internal medicine and geriatric medicine. He practiced for 14 years in a small Minnesota town, and is now practicing general internal medicine at the Olmsted Medical Group in Rochester, Minnesota. He and his wife, Barbara Yawn, MD, publish a monthly newsletter for rural physicians.